# CRNA
## Exam
### Part 2 of 2

# SECRETS

## Study Guide
### Your Key to Exam Success

CRNA Test Review for the Certified
Registered Nurse Anesthetist Exam

Dear Future Exam Success Story:

First of all, **THANK YOU** for purchasing Mometrix study materials!

Second, congratulations! You are one of the few determined test-takers who are committed to doing whatever it takes to excel on your exam. **You have come to the right place.** We developed these study materials with one goal in mind: to deliver you the information you need in a format that's concise and easy to use.

In addition to optimizing your guide for the content of the test, we've outlined our recommended steps for breaking down the preparation process into small, attainable goals so you can make sure you stay on track.

We've also analyzed the entire test-taking process, identifying the most common pitfalls and showing how you can overcome them and be ready for any curveball the test throws you.

Standardized testing is one of the biggest obstacles on your road to success, which only increases the importance of doing well in the high-pressure, high-stakes environment of test day. Your results on this test could have a significant impact on your future, and this guide provides the information and practical advice to help you achieve your full potential on test day.

### Your success is our success

**We would love to hear from you!** If you would like to share the story of your exam success or if you have any questions or comments in regard to our products, please contact us at **800-673-8175** or **support@mometrix.com**.

Thanks again for your business and we wish you continued success!

Sincerely,
The Mometrix Test Preparation Team


**Need more help? Check out our flashcards at:** http://MometrixFlashcards.com/CRNA

# TABLE OF CONTENTS

BASIC PRINCIPLES OF ANESTHESIA (CONTINUED) ...................................................................... 1
   LOCAL/REGIONAL ANESTHETICS ........................................................................................ 1
   MONITORED ANESTHESIA CARE ...................................................................................... 12
   PAIN MANAGEMENT .......................................................................................................... 13
   OTHER TECHNIQUES ........................................................................................................ 18
   POSTANESTHESIA CARE/RESPIRATORY CARE ................................................................. 19
   PAIN THEORY .................................................................................................................. 21

ADVANCED PRINCIPLES OF ANESTHESIA ................................................................................ 23
   SURGICAL PROCEDURES AND PROCEDURES RELATED TO ORGAN SYSTEMS ..................... 23
   PEDIATRICS ..................................................................................................................... 83
   OBSTETRICS ..................................................................................................................... 94
   GERIATRICS ................................................................................................................... 102

PROFESSIONAL ISSUES .......................................................................................................... 105

CRNA PRACTICE TEST ......................................................................................................... 111

ANSWER KEY AND EXPLANATIONS ........................................................................................ 122

HOW TO OVERCOME TEST ANXIETY ...................................................................................... 126
   CAUSES OF TEST ANXIETY .............................................................................................. 126
   ELEMENTS OF TEST ANXIETY .......................................................................................... 127
   EFFECTS OF TEST ANXIETY ............................................................................................. 127
   PHYSICAL STEPS FOR BEATING TEST ANXIETY ............................................................... 128
   MENTAL STEPS FOR BEATING TEST ANXIETY .................................................................. 129
   STUDY STRATEGY .......................................................................................................... 130
   TEST TIPS ...................................................................................................................... 132
   IMPORTANT QUALIFICATION ........................................................................................... 133

THANK YOU ........................................................................................................................... 134

ADDITIONAL BONUS MATERIAL ............................................................................................. 135

# Basic Principles of Anesthesia (continued)

## Local/Regional Anesthetics

### Local anesthesia

Local anesthesia (removing the sensation of pain without affecting the level of consciousness) is anesthesia of a small portion of the body, such as the area of a tooth, a finger, or tissue around a small laceration. Regional anesthesia encompasses a larger area, such as a limb. **Infiltration** is a type of local anesthesia in which an anesthetic solution is injected directly into the tissue adjacent to cutaneous nerves. **Field block** is a type of infiltration block that causes anesthesia distal to the infiltration. Local anesthetics (prilocaine, mepivacaine, bupivacaine, and ropivacaine) block sodium channels, inhibiting conduction by preventing sodium ions from entering a neuron and potassium ions from leaving. Thick myelinated nerve fibers are more resistive to local anesthetics than thin demyelinated nerves; this difference affects the amount and type of anesthetic agent used. Epinephrine may be added to the anesthetic to produce vasoconstriction and prevent absorption of the anesthetic agent away from the site of injection. Central nervous system and cardiovascular complications can occur with toxic levels of anesthetic agents.

### Potency of local anesthetic agents

**Potency** of a local anesthetic relates to the following:

- *Lipid solubility:* Increased levels correlate with greater potency.
- *Protein binding ability:* Increased ability correlates with longer duration of action.
- *Acid dissociation constant ($pK_a$):* Relates to the nonionized lipid-soluble fraction of an anesthetic agent that can cross the nephron membrane. It indicates the degree of acidity: agents with a $pK_a$ closest to normal pH (7.4) usually have a faster onset of action. All local anesthetics have a higher pH (less acidic); therefore, a higher $pK_a$ delays onset (except for chloroprocaine because of its increased concentration). Because most local anesthetic agents have a $pK_a$ of less than 8, onset is within 2 to 4 minutes. Agents with $pK_a$ higher than 8 include bupivacaine (8.1), which has an onset of 5 to 8 minutes (but its 96% protein binding provides a long duration of action), and procaine (9.1), which has an onset of 14 to 18 minutes (but 6% protein binding renders it very short-acting).

The absorption rate may be affected by tissue changes (increased tissue acidity with infection), vascularity, rate of administration, and total dose.

### Locating peripheral nerves

There are 3 primary methods of **locating peripheral nerves** for injection of local anesthetics:

- *Paresthesia:* This is a radiating electric-like sensation that occurs when the needle is in close proximity to a nerve. This sensation can indicate intraneural placement and should not be purposely elicited. Intraneural administration can cause ischemia to the nerve and permanent damage; therefore, if persistent paresthesia or severe pain occurs, the needle should be repositioned. A blunt beveled needle is often used because the blunt tip tends to push the nerve aside rather than penetrate it.

- **Nerve stimulation:** A low-output nerve stimulator attached to a special insulation-coated needle (cathode) elicits an electrical current (≤0.5 mA) that is detected by a lead on the body (anode). Muscle contractions increase in proximity to the nerve and decrease as the needle moves away. The Raj test (injection of 1-2 mL local anesthetic) should eliminate the motor response.
- **Ultrasonography** (high-resolution): Imaging allows direct visualization of nerves and other structures, needle placement, and distribution of agent.

Currently no technique has been shown to have more favorable outcomes or less side effects or complications than another.

### Intercostobrachial, medial brachial, and intercostal blocks

A number of **regional nerve blocks** are used as adjuncts to other blocks or to relieve pain:

- **Intercostobrachial** (from T2) and **medial brachial** (from C8 and T1) cutaneous nerves: A field block is used to block these nerves at the humeral head (pectoral ridge), where they are superficial. Both are blocked proximal to the axilla for procedures involving the shoulder or for other surgical procedures to the arm that require a pneumatic tourniquet.
- **Intercostal block:** These blocks are usually used for intercostal nerves between the sixth and eleventh ribs, because the nerves are easily palpable. Intercostal blocks can provide sensory and motor anesthesia for the chest wall. Anesthesia is not generally sufficient for surgery, but the blocks may be used to reduce pain after rib fractures or to reduce postsurgical pain after breast or thoracic surgery.

### Topical

**Topical anesthetics**, such as EMLA (eucharistic mixture of local anesthetics) cream, composed of 2.5% lidocaine and 2.5% prilocaine, or topical sprays have limited surgical use and are primarily used to reduce pain and itching or to prevent pain. They may be administered before venipuncture, intramuscular injections, or even injection for local anesthesia. EMLA, the most frequently used, must be applied to intact skin. It may be used for simple skin biopsies; however, because it must be applied 60 to 90 minutes before the procedure with an occlusive dressing for optimal effectiveness, its use is limited. A newer preparation, ELA-Max (available in both 4% and 5% lidocaine), is effective within 30 to 40 minutes and does not require an occlusive dressing. These preparations should be considered for use with pediatric patients or with adults who have "needle phobia." ELA-Max is safer for neonates because it does not contain prilocaine, which can in rare circumstances cause methemoglobinemia.

### Anatomic considerations for neuraxial anesthesia

**Neuraxial anesthesia** requires an understanding of spinal anatomy and physiology:

- **Vertebral column** (spine): Comprised of 7 cervical, 12 thoracic, and 5 vertebrae connected by cushioning intervertebral disks and supported by ligaments. The sacrum is a fusion of 5 sacral vertebrae, with an opening called the sacral hiatus between the fourth and fifth sacral vertebrae (fused in 8% of adults). The vertebral column surrounds and protects the spinal cord and nerve roots. Cervical nerves exit the vertebral column superior to the corresponding vertebrae, but at the first thoracic vertebra (T1) the nerves exit inferior to the corresponding vertebrae, resulting in 8 cervical nerve roots but only 7 cervical vertebrae.

- ***Spinal cord:*** Begins at the rostral border of the medulla and extends to L3 in the infant (<1 year) but to L1 in children and adults, with a depth of 1 to 1.5 cm in the infant and 3 to 4 cm in the adult. The nerves continue below the spine in the cauda equina until they exit the intervertebral foramen in the lower lumbar or sacral area. The spinal cord contains the cerebrospinal fluid and is covered by 3 protective membranes (meninges) that are continuous around the brain and spinal cord:
- ***Pia mater***, the innermost layer, adheres to the spinal cord.
- ***Subarachnoid space*** between the pia mater and arachnoid mater (the next layer) contains the cerebrospinal fluid. Spinal (subarachnoid) anesthesia is administered into this space.
- ***Arachnoid mater*** is the primary impermeable barrier preventing movement of drugs from the epidural to the subarachnoid space. It is closely adherent to the dura mater (outside layer)
- ***Dura mater*** is a protective fibroelastic membrane that is fairly impenetrable.
- ***Epidural space*** lies outside the dura mater and contains lymphatics, fatty tissue, nerve roots, small arteries, and the epidural venous plexus. Epidural and caudal anesthesia is administered into this space. The (adult) depth ranges from 6 mm at L2 to 4 or 5 mm in the midthoracic area.

**Subarachnoid block**

A **subarachnoid (spinal) block** is begun after an intravenous infusion has been started. An opioid may be given to decrease discomfort and local infiltration at the insertion point. The spine should be flexed to increase the interspinous space. Positions include the following:

- ***Lateral***: This position is most comfortable for those who are very ill or frail and allows for higher levels of sedation.
- ***Sitting***: This facilitates insertion of the needle and favors a caudal distribution but cannot be used with heavy sedation and may cause vasovagal syncope.
- ***Prone***: This is a difficult position for insertion and monitoring and is rarely used except for some perianal surgical procedures in which the patient is in the jackknife position.

Because the spinal cord descends to L3 in about 2% of adults, the point of insertion should not be above L3 or L4 so that spinal trauma can be avoided. The approach may be midline or paramedian (approximately 1 cm lateral to the midline).

The needle is advanced through the dura (pop felt) and into the subarachnoid space. After insertion into the subarachnoid space, the needle should be advanced slightly. CSF flow indicates correct placement of the needle. If CSF remains blood-tinged, reinsertion is required. Once the syringe has been attached to the needle, aspiration is performed to ensure proper placement. The anesthetic agent is injected over 3 to 5 seconds, followed by slight aspiration and reinjection to verify correct delivery. The needle is withdrawn, and the patient is placed in the position needed for correct distribution. Distribution is affected by the volume of anesthetic, the rate of injection, anatomical features (such as size of subarachnoid space), gravity (position of patient), and baricity (related to density of CSF). Catheters may be used for administration of continuous spinal anesthesia, allowing repeated administration for prolonged procedures, but catheters should inserted only 2 to 4 cm to avoid spinal trauma. Sympathetic blockade is 2 levels above sensory blockade.

## Baricity related to subarachnoid blocks

**Baricity** is the density of anesthetic agent compared to that of CSF:

- ***Hyperbaric solutions:*** Contain glucose to increase baricity. They allow for cephalad spread. The horizontal supine position distributes to T6, and the Trendelenburg position increases distribution for abdominal surgery. If administered caudad to the lumbosacral peak, distribution is restricted to the "saddle block" area. Because placing the patient in the lateral position reduces flow caused by spinal curve, distribution is controlled by the position of the operating table (head up, level, or head down).
- ***Hypobaric solutions:*** Contain sterile water or sterile saline to decrease baricity. These solutions are rarely used except when the patient is in the jackknife position, in which case the distribution should "float" upward to the nondependent area.
- ***Isobaric solutions:*** Usually contain sterile saline. These tend to have little distribution (unaffected by gravity) and remain near the injection site. They also produce more motor block and a longer duration of action than hyperbaric solutions. Isobaric solutions are used for perineal procedures or procedures on the lower extremities and the lower trunk (hip surgery or hernia repair).

## Complications related to subarachnoid block

A number of complications are related to **subarachnoid block:**

- ***Cardiovascular***: Hypotension lower than 90 mm Hg systolic is the most common occurrence (affecting approximately 33% of patients) and may be associated with bradycardia (affecting approximately 10% to 15%) and a decrease in contractility. Blocking sympathetic fibers at T5-L1 may cause vasodilation and decreases in venous return and cardiac output, minimized by compensatory vasoconstriction above the area of the block. Hypotension may be avoided with volume loading of 10 to 20 mL/kg of IV fluid. The Trendelenburg position at 5° to 10° may relieve symptoms. Direct α-agonists (phenylephrine) and ephedrine may be used as treatment with epinephrine (1.0 mg IV) for profound bradycardia or asystole.
- ***Respiratory***: Complications are usually minimal because diaphragmatic innervation is at the level of C3 to C6; however, patients with COPD, who use intercostal and abdominal muscles to assist respirations, may suffer respiratory distress. Surgery of the thoracic area or upper abdominal area may be associated with hypoventilation, atelectasis, and difficulty coughing to clear airway. Total spinal anesthesia may cause apnea.
- ***High or total (excessive) spinal anesthesia***: This excess of sensory and motor anesthesia results in loss of consciousness and may precipitate severe hypotension and apnea. Symptoms usually manifest themselves rapidly. Treatment includes the Trendelenburg position (reverse Trendelenburg should not be used because of possible compromise of cerebral blood flow). Tracheal intubation is usually required, especially for those at risk (such as pregnant women), and may require an IV induction agent.
- ***Gastrointestinal:*** Nausea, vomiting, and decreased gastric motility may occur, often related to hypotension.
- ***Urinary***: Bladder retention may occur because nerves that innervate the bladder are blocked. Urinary catheterization may be necessary.
- ***Back pain***: Back pain near the injection site is common and usually transient. It may relate to multiple punctures or position.

- **Neurological**: Trauma to the spinal cord may occur directly from needle or catheter insertion or indirectly from resultant hematoma or infection. Transient paresis may occur, especially with lidocaine administration. Administration of an anesthetic agent in the presence of paresthesia increases the risk of permanent neurological compromise; therefore, administration should be discontinued if paresthesia occurs. Postdural puncture headache results from loss of CSF through a puncture hole in the dura, resulting in displacement of the brain posteriorly and stress on supporting structures. Onset of headache is 12 to 48 hours after puncture but may be delayed for weeks or months in some cases. Headache (frontal, occipital, or both) is usually intensified by sitting or standing and may be dull or throbbing and accompanied by GI upset or ocular disturbances. Treatment is usually conservative (bed rest, fluids, caffeine); alternatively, an autologous blood patch (15 to 20 mL) may be injected epidurally near the puncture site.

## Epidural block

**Epidural blocks**, often used for labor and birth, can be performed at the lumbar, thoracic, or cervical level for either anesthesia or analgesia with a single administration or continuous administration via catheter. The height and duration of the blockade and presence or absence of motor blockade depend on the anesthetic agent, the concentration and dosage, the site of injection, the patient's age and weight, and the use or non-use of a vasoconstrictor. Epidural onset (10-20 minutes) is slower than subarachnoid onset and requires a larger volume of anesthetic agent (15-20 mL). The most common insertion site is L1-L5, usually using a midline (most common) or paramedian approach, with care taken not to pierce the dura. This block is adequate for procedures below the diaphragm. If a catheter is used, it is threaded 3 to 5 cm into the epidural space; aspiration is used to ensure that there is no return of CSF or blood, and a test dose is given. Thoracic and cervical blocks are used primarily for analgesia.

## Techniques for ensuring proper epidural placement

Two techniques can be used to determine correct **placement** of the needle or catheter into the epidural space:

- **Loss-of-resistance technique:** A needle (attached to a syringe containing saline, air, or both) is advanced while resistance to injection is assessed. If the needle is within the ligamentum flavum, the plunger springs back. The resistance drops abruptly as the needle is advanced into the epidural space and saline is injected.
- **Hanging-drop technique:** A small drop of saline is placed at the distal end of the needle; as the needle passes through the ligamentum flavum; negative pressure forces the saline back into the needle. This method is less reliable than the loss-of-resistance technique.

A **test dose** of anesthetic (3 mL lidocaine 1.5% with 1:200,000 epinephrine or 3 mL 2% lidocaine) is injected into the epidural space to ensure proper placement. The patient is observed for 3 to 5 minutes for indications of intravascular (tachycardia, increased BP, tremor) or intrathecal placement (evidence of spinal anesthesia, hypotension, respiratory depression). This method is less reliable with the elderly than with younger patients.

## Use of adjuvants subarachnoid and epidural blocks

**Adjuvants** may be added to the anesthetic agents for subarachnoid and epidural blocks:

- *Epinephrine*: Vasoconstrictors increase the duration of spinal anesthesia by decreasing cord blood flow. It is more effective with tetracaine and bupivacaine than lidocaine. There is some indication that using epinephrine and lidocaine may increase lidocaine neurotoxicity. For epidurals, this vasoconstrictor reduces vascular absorption of the anesthetic agent from the epidural space, prolonging the duration of anesthesia and reducing systemic toxicity. This is more effective with lidocaine or chloroprocaine than with bupivacaine.
- *Opioids*: Opioids, such as fentanyl, may be used for short-duration spinal anesthesia, but longer-acting morphine requires monitoring for respiratory depression. For epidurals, lipid solubility is more important. Lipophilic opioids (fentanyl) are rapidly absorbed systemically, but hydrophilic opioids (morphine) spread rostrally within the CSF.
- *Sodium bicarbonate:* Used for epidurals, alkalinization promotes a more rapid onset of anesthesia. It should not be used with bupivacaine, which precipitates an alkaline pH.

## Complications of epidural blocks

A number of **complications** are associated with **epidural blocks:**

- *Hypotension* may occur because of sympathetic nervous system block, but it is less common and less pronounced than with subarachnoid block.
- *Intravascular injection* can result in systemic absorption. This rarely causes severe problems, especially with epinephrine, but some evidence of toxicity (restlessness, slurring speech, and tinnitus) may occur and in rare cases may be life threatening. Cardiac toxicity is associated with bupivacaine.
- *Subarachnoid injection* may cause rapid total spinal anesthesia because of the larger volume of anesthetic agent used for epidurals. This can result in permanent neurological damage. Therefore, accidental injection into the subarachnoid space may require irrigation with saline if CSF can be readily aspirated. A dilated nonreactive pupil may indicate intrathecal injection.
- *Subdural injection* produces an unusual irregular block and poses the danger of piercing into the subarachnoid space.
- *Neural damage* can occur during this procedure, especially if paresthesia occurs during the procedure. Most paresthesia is transient.

## Caudal block

The **caudal block** is a type of epidural block into the sacral portion of the epidural space. This block is used frequently for pediatric surgery (urogenital, rectal, inguinal, lower extremity), combined with general anesthesia, and for anorectal surgery for adults. It is also used for acute and chronic pain control. Administration is through the sacral hiatus between S4 and S5. If this area is fused (sacralization) in adults, then this procedure may be impossible. Administration requires that children be placed in the prone or lateral position with hips flexed and that adults be placed in the prone, lateral, or jackknife position. The needle is inserted through the sacrococcygeal ligament at a 60° to 90° angle and then redirected upward, penetrating 1 to 2 mm within the spinal canal. Placement is confirmed by rapidly injecting air or saline while palpating the tissue below the caudal canal for swelling, which indicates incorrect placement. Subarachnoid injection may occur if the needle is advanced too far.

## Combined spinal and epidural

Both spinal anesthesia and an epidural catheter may be placed at the same time for **combined subarachnoid and epidural anesthesia**. This combined anesthesia has the advantage of rapid onset (from the subarachnoid injection) and extended duration (from the epidural). This combination is frequently used with obstetric and orthopedic procedures (such as hip or knee replacement). The procedure involves placement of an epidural needle and passage of a small spinal needle through the lumen of the epidural needle into the subarachnoid space. The spinal anesthetic agent is administered first and the needle is removed. Then the epidural catheter is advanced into the epidural space. Commercially available combined needles may be used. There is some concern that the subarachnoid puncture site may allow leakage of a large volume of anesthetic agent into the subarachnoid space.

## Brachial plexus block

- *Infraclavicular block* for surgery of the upper arm, forearm, and elbow or placement of catheter for postoperative pain management. Complications are more likely than with supraclavicular block and include pneumothorax, hemothorax, and (with left-sided block) chylothorax (presence of diffused chyle in the pleural cavity).
- *Interscalene block* for surgery of the shoulder, arm, and elbow. It is less effective for procedures affecting the ulnar nerve distribution. Complications include block of phrenic nerve with respiratory failure, Horner's syndrome, dyspnea, and hoarseness. Seizure can occur if anesthetic is injected into the vertebral artery. Pneumothorax can occur if the pleura is punctured.
- *Supraclavicular block* for surgery of the entire arm, including the hand. Complications include a high incidence of pneumothorax ($\leq 6\%$). Horner's syndrome (myosis, ptosis, and anhidrosis) and block of the phrenic nerve with respiratory failure can occur.

The brachial plexus is a nerve plexus originating from the ventral branches of the last four cervical (C4-C8) and the first thoracic (T1-T2) spinal nerves, giving off many of the principal nerves of the shoulder, chest, and arms. Because the brachial plexus is encased in a sheath, injection into any point in the sheath spreads the block to C5-T1, although the extent of block varies with the level of injection. Sometimes additional nerves must be blocked separately. The **brachial plexus block** may be administered according to surgical site:

- *Axillary block* for surgery of the forearm and hand, along the ulnar nerve distribution. This approach may miss the medial brachial cutaneous nerve, which may leave the sheath below the clavicle. Complications are rare if the block is administered properly and intravascular administration is avoided.
- *Midhumeral block* allows for blocking of the 4 major nerves of the arm separately and is used for surgery of the forearm and hand (similar to axillary). This block is similar to the axillary block in success, but the onset is slower.

## Airway blocks (glossopharyngeal)

**Airway blocks** are typically used in conjunction with awake intubation to remove the gag and coughing reflex and facilitate placement. A number of methods may be used to provide anesthesia:

- *Glossopharyngeal:* The glossopharyngeal nerve (cranial IX) innervates the posterior tongue, oropharynx, soft palate, tonsils, and epiglottis (pharyngeal surface). A glossopharyngeal block eliminates the gag reflex and facilitates intubation. The block may be done through the open mouth by applying topical anesthetic to the tongue and then injecting an anesthetic agent (approximately 5 mL) into the submucosa at the palatopharyngeal fold. Alternatively, the block may be performed with the patient lying supine and the nerve accessed externally at the styloid process between the mandible and the mastoid process. Intravascular injection is possible with both approaches (the carotid artery is adjacent); therefore, careful administration with aspiration is necessary. Epinephrine may be added to decrease absorption in this vascular area. The glossopharyngeal nerve block alone is not adequate for intubation but is used as part of the airway anesthesia.
- *Topical:* Spray anesthetics may be applied directly to mucous membranes in the nose or mouth. Another choice is anesthetic solution applied to a cotton pledget that is then placed in a specific area, such as the nares, for 10 to 15 minutes. In some cases, a mouth swish may provide adequate topical anesthesia. Topical anesthesia can also be applied via a nebulizer (lidocaine 2-4%) with a mouthpiece or facemask to aerosolize anesthetic solution, although this method requires about 30 minutes for effective anesthesia. The primary problem with inhalation is that results are variable and the cough reflex may persist. Epinephrine added to the anesthetic agent can reduce bleeding during intubation.
- *Recurrent laryngeal block:* This block prevents the cough reflex while the intubation tube is passing through the vocal chords. The recurrent laryngeal nerve is a branch of the vagus (cranial X) nerve and innervates the vocal folds and trachea. This block may be administered effectively by inhalational anesthesia for some patients. However, a transtracheal block may be necessary for others. With the patient in the supine position and the neck extended, the cricothyroid membrane is identified and the subcutaneous tissue at the site is anesthetized with local infiltration before the needle is inserted perpendicular to the trachea. Aspiration is performed continuously until loss of negative pressure indicates that the needle has entered the larynx. Injecting the anesthetic agent triggers cough, which helps to distribute the agent. In some cases, this area may be anesthetized directly through the fiberoptic bronchoscope by spraying anesthetic agent through the injection port.
- *Superior laryngeal nerve block:* The superior laryngeal nerve is a branch of the vagus nerve (cranial X). The internal branch innervates the tongue (base), epiglottis, and mucous membranes of the pharynx above the vocal chords. Block may use topical or inhaled anesthetics, but these do not always provide reliable anesthesia and may be too time-consuming. Direct regional block may be administered through bilateral injections at the hyoid bone (greater cornu) below the mandible while the patient is in the supine position with the neck extended. Block may also be administered in the pre-epiglottic space, lateral to the thyroid notch. Care must be taken to avoid the carotid artery. If patients cannot tolerate injections, the block may be performed after application of a topical spray with anesthetic-soaked pledgets placed bilaterally at the pyriform fossae at the tongue root for 5 to 10 minutes. This procedure is used in conjunction with other blocks for intubation.

- *Palatine nerve block:* The palatine nerves (most originating from the maxillary nerve) innervate the nasal cavities, including the turbinates and 66% of the nasal septum (posterior aspect). This nerve block is often successful with a topical anesthetic applied inside the nasal passages. Another topical technique involves soaking a cotton applicator in anesthetic agent and passing it along the upper aspect of the middle turbinate to the back of the nasopharynx, leaving it in contact with the posterior wall for approximately 20 minutes. This method effectively blocks the pterygopalatine ganglion from which the nerves are derived. This ganglion may also be injected with anesthetic agent through the open mouth into the pterygopalatine fossa. The ganglion may also be accessed percutaneously via the mandibular notch, but this procedure is usually performed under fluoroscopic guidance as part of pain management. There is a high risk of vascular injection. The injectable techniques are rarely used because of the difficulty of obtaining access.

## Facial nerve block

A **facial nerve block** is often used to supplement a retrobulbar block to prevent squinting of the eyelids and allow placement of a lid speculum. Local infiltration to block the orbicularis oculi muscle or a block of the branches of the facial nerve can be done to effect motor anesthesia. The block can be performed by using several approaches:

- *Van Lint:* The block requires subcutaneous injection of an anesthetic agent at the outer canthus of the eye, directed toward the eyebrow and the infraorbital foramen. This blocks the temporal division of the facial nerve.
- *Atkinson:* This block is done at the zygomatic arch, where the facial nerve crosses.
- *O'Brien:* This block is done at the mandibular condyle, below the posterior zygomatic process.
- *Nadbath*: This block affects the facial nerve at the stylomastoid foramen under the auditory canal. It is not recommended because of serious complications, such as vocal cord paralysis, difficulty in swallowing, and respiratory distress.

## Retrobulbar and peribulbar block

**Retrobulbar** and **peribulbar blocks** are used to provide regional anesthesia for intraocular and orbital surgery lasting no longer than 2 hours, including procedures involving the cornea, anterior chamber, and lens. Usually a combination of lidocaine and bupivacaine is used for both blocks. Epinephrine may be added to prolong anesthesia, and hyaluronidase may be added to enhance the distribution. Because the patient must be able to cooperate, these blocks are used for adults:

- *Retrobulbar*: The needle is inserted below the eye and punctures the bulbar fascia, entering the orbital muscle cone. A small volume (2-4 mL) of anesthetic agent is used with onset in 2 minutes. Motor block of eyelid may require additional block of cranial verve VI.
- *Peribulbar:* The needle is inserted through the lower lid, just above the inferior orbital rim toward the orbit, penetrating the lower orbital septum, parallel and lateral to the bulbar fascia. A larger volume (4-12 mL) of anesthetic agent is used with onset in 10 to 20 minutes. The danger of complications is reduced, but the block may cause conjunctival edema.

## Digital block

Four small digital nerves innervate each finger, entering at the base with 2 on the dorsolateral surface (small nerves enervating the back of the fingers to the first joint) and 2 on the ventrolateral surface (the main nerves), distributed at the 4 corners. **Digital block** is performed for surgery on the fingers. Epinephrine should never be used in digital nerve blocks because of the potential for tissue damage due to vasoconstriction. Injection may be made into each side of the base of the finger. A transthecal digital block (injecting into the flexor tendon sheath) allows a block with only one injection for the digit rather than two injections. With digital blocks, discomfort is reduced by performing small local surface infiltration before the needle is advanced for the digital block. Complications include intraneural or intravascular administration of anesthetic agent.

### Ankle block

An **ankle block** includes 5 separate blocks. Four nerves are branches of the sciatic nerve:

- Deep peroneal (enervating the webbing between the first and second toes).
- Superficial peroneal (enervating the dorsum of the foot).
- Tibial (enervating the sole of the foot).
- Sural (enervating the lateral side of the foot).

The fourth nerve is a branch of the femoral nerve:

- Saphenous nerve (enervating the medial aspect of the foot), a branch of the femoral nerve.

The ankle block, performed at the level of the malleoli, is used for podiatric surgery and amputation or debridement of the foot or toes. The anesthetic agent should never contain epinephrine. The relatively poor blood supply usually precludes systemic toxicity. The block, administered at the ankle, anesthetizes the foot but not the ankle itself. The patient is in the supine position with the foot supported on a block to allow access to all sites for blocking.

### Ilioinguinal and iliohypogastric nerve blocks

The lumbar plexus is formed by the ventral branches of the second to the fifth lumbar nerves in the psoas major muscle (the branches of the first lumbar nerve are often included). Terminal branches of the lumbar plexus include the ilioinguinal nerve (enervating the scrotum and penis in males and part of labia and mons pubis in females) and the iliohypogastric nerve (enervating the anterolateral gluteal region) with some fibers from L1 and T12. Together they innervate abdominal muscles and the inguinal canal. An **ilioinguinal and iliohypogastric block** is used for surgery of the inguinal and genital regions, such as herniorrhaphy. To provide adequate analgesia, blockade should be administered both between the transversus abdominus and internal oblique muscles and between the internal oblique and external oblique muscles. This is a common block for hernia repairs in infants and children, often facilitated by ultrasound guidance, but it is less commonly used for adults, who generally are given general anesthesia.

### IV regional (Bier) block

An intravenous regional block (**Bier block**) is most commonly used for surgery on the forearm (wrist) and hand, including the digits. With this block, circulation is occluded by a tourniquet (Esmarch bandage inflated to 100 mm Hg above patient's systolic BP), and a solution is administered through an intravenous catheter placed in the distal limb. Bier block is most effective for procedures lasting less than 1 or 2 hours because severe pain is associated with tourniquet use after approximately 45 minutes. Commonly used agents include 15 to 50 mL of 0.5% to 2% lidocaine solutions without epinephrine. Ropivacaine (1.2-1.8 mg/kg in 40 mL) or 40 mL of 0.125% levobupivacaine may be used for adults if there is concern about cardiovascular or central nervous system toxicity that may occur after the tourniquet is released. The duration of action directly relates to the time of inflation of the tourniquet. The use of a double tourniquet with alternating

- 10 -

inflation or blockade of the intercostobrachial nerve by infiltration may be used to reduce tourniquet pain.

## Wrist block

**Wrist block** may be used for surgery on the hand (if pneumatic tourniquet is not used) or to supplement a brachial plexus block that lacks complete sensory distribution. Blockade can be done at the elbow, but results are not significantly different than when done at the wrist. These blocks are indicated for carpal tunnel, hand, or finger surgery. Complications include intravascular or intraneural administration of anesthetic agent. The radial nerve, ulnar nerve, and median nerve share innervation of the hand. Blocks include the following:

- *Radial nerve block:* Anesthetizes the dorsal aspects of the hand (radial side). This block frequently supplements a brachial plexus block.
- *Ulnar nerve block:* Anesthetizes the dorsal and palmar surfaces of the ulnar aspect of the hand. This block may be used alone for minor hand procedures (ulnar distribution) or as a supplement to axillary or interscalene block.
- *Median nerve block:* Anesthetizes the palmar surface of the hand (radial side). This block is almost always used as a supplement to brachial plexus block.

## Femoral block

The femoral nerve, originating in the lumbar plexus (L2-L4), innervates the anterior thigh and knee:

- *Femoral block:* Useful for superficial procedures, such as muscle biopsy, skin grafting, knee arthroscopy, and patellar surgery. It is often combined with other blocks (such as sciatic) for surgical procedures of the knee or anterior thigh (such as quadriceps tendon repair) or for postoperative control of pain. Administration is at a point 2 cm lateral to the femoral artery pulse and 2 cm distal to the inguinal line (connecting the anterior superior iliac spine and the superior-lateral corner of the pubic tubercle). This block is also referred to as the "3-in-1 block" because it may also block the obturator and lateral femoral cutaneous nerves. An indwelling catheter may be put in place for continuous perineural infusion (often in conjunction with sciatic nerve block) to reduce pain after total knee arthroplasty.

## Sciatic block

The sciatic nerve originates within the sacral plexus (L4-5, S1-3). The sciatic nerve is large (2 cm) as it exits the pelvis and travels down the buttocks and the posterior aspect of the leg. **Sciatic block** is used for pain control and for surgical procedures on the knee, calf, tibia, ankle (including the Achilles tendon), and foot:

- *Sciatic nerve block:* This block provides almost complete anesthesia of the lower limb except for the anteromedial aspect (innervated by the saphenous nerve). Sedation is required because of discomfort during the block. Block is administered with the patient in the lateral decubitus position. The needle insertion point is 4 cm perpendicular and caudal to the midpoint of a line between the grater trochanter and the posterior-superior iliac spine. Anesthetic agent is chosen on the basis of the length of the surgical procedure. Epinephrine should not be used because it may increase ischemia. Insertion is guided by nerve stimulation. This block may be combined with a femoral or lumbar plexus block.

## Popliteal block

The **popliteal nerve block** is given proximal to the point at which the sciatic nerve divides into the peroneal and tibial nerves at the popliteal fossa. Ultrasound is useful for guidance because there is variability in the point of division. There are 3 approaches:

- *Posterior intertendinous block:* This block is performed with the patient in the prone position. It provides anesthesia of the distal two-thirds of the lower limb (except for the medial aspect). It is used for surgery of the ankle or foot, such as debridement or repair of the Achilles tendon.
- *Lateral block:* This block is performed with the patient in the lateral position. It provides anesthesia in a distribution similar to that provided by the posterior intertendinous block. The lateral block is used for surgery on the calf, ankle (including Achilles tendon), and foot and provides anesthesia for use of the calf tourniquet.
- *Supine (lithotomy) block:* This block is performed with the patient's leg supported for access to the popliteal fossa. Distribution and use are similar to those of other approaches, but this block can be used if the lateral or prone position is problematic.

## Lateral femoral cutaneous block, saphenous block

The femoral nerve gives rise to lateral cutaneous nerves from the anterior division (enervating the lateral aspect of the thighs) and to the saphenous nerve from the posterior division (enervating the medial aspect of the leg distal to the knee):

- *Lateral femoral cutaneous block:* This block is useful for superficial procedures, such as biopsies or skin grafts, but is used with other blocks for surgery on or proximal to the knee. The administration site is 2 cm distal and 2cm medial to the anterior iliac spine and through the fascia lata.
- *Saphenous block:* This block is used most commonly with a sciatic or popliteal block as a supplement for vascular, orthopedic, or podiatric procedures of the lower leg. For foot surgery, the block is administered at the medial malleolus. Generally, low volume femoral block is effective for blocking the saphenous nerve.

# Monitored Anesthesia Care

## Conscious sedation

**Conscious sedation** is used to decrease sensations of pain and awareness caused by a surgical or invasive procedure, such as breast biopsy, vasectomy, fracture repair, endoscopy, and dental procedures. It is also used during presurgical preparations, such as insertion of central lines, catheters, and use of cooling blankets. Conscious sedation uses a combination of analgesia and sedation so that patients can remain responsive and follow verbal cues but have brief amnesia preventing recall of the procedures. Careful monitoring, including pulse oximetry, is necessary during this type of sedation.

The most commonly used drugs include the following:

- Midazolam (Versed): This is a short-acting water-soluble sedative, with an onset of 1 to 5 minutes, a peak at 30 minutes, and duration of approximately 1 hour (but may last for up to 6 hours).
- Fentanyl: This is a short-acting opioid with immediate onset, a peak at 10 to 15 minutes, and duration of approximately 20 to 45 minutes.

The fentanyl/midazolam combination provides both sedation and pain control. Conscious sedation usually requires that the patient fast for 6 hours before administration.

# Pain Management

## Epidural analgesia (opioids)

**Epidural analgesia** with opioids is a common method of postoperative pain management, but its onset of action is often 3 to 4 hours. The opioid is administered into the epidural space, but to contact the opioid receptors of the substantia gelatinosa of the spinal cord it must cross the dura. Its distribution is slowed further by fat and connective tissue in the epidural area. Additionally, much of the opioid may be absorbed systemically because the area is vascular and the dosage must be approximately 10 times higher than for intrathecal administration; this systemic absorption sometimes causes systemic depression. Sometimes an initial bolus of medication is given along with a local anesthetic to block the transmission of pain and overcome the delay in onset. Both long-acting and short-acting opioids may be used together:

- *Hydrophilic opioids* (such as morphine) tend to spread rostrally with CSF along the entire spinal cord; therefore, they can be given at a lower level and still provide relief at a higher level.
- *Lipophilic opioids* (such as fentanyl) tend to provide more segmental relief with less distribution.

## Epidural steroids

**Epidural steroids** are administered for back pain related to neural compression. They are most effective if given within 2 weeks of pain onset. Medications include the following:

- Methylprednisolone acetate (40-80 mg).
- Triamcinolone diacetate (40-80 mg).

*[handwritten: application of methylprednisolone was found to reversibly block transmission in the unmyelinated C fibers but not in the A & B fibers]*

The medication may be administered with saline or a small amount of local anesthetic agent. The needle must be flushed before it is removed so that steroids do not create a fistula. The antiinflammatory response usually takes effect within 12 to 48 hours, reducing pain. One dose is often sufficient, although if pain persists, the treatment may be repeated. Serial treatments are avoided because of the potential for adrenal suppression. Needle insertion may be performed under fluoroscopic guidance to prevent inadvertent intravascular, subdural, or subarachnoid administration. The epidural may be translaminar or transforaminal (targeting selective nerve roots). Most injections are given in the lumbar area. Caudal administration may be used if there is scarring from previous surgery, although there may be less-than-adequate migration to the site of injury.

## Somatic and sympathetic nerve blocks

**Somatic** nerves leave the spinal column as nerve roots and may form a plexus or an individual nerve. Plexi include cervical, brachial, lumbosacral, and sacral. Individual nerves include the occipital, intercostal, and suprascapular. Somatic nerve blocks are used for both acute and chronic pain and for postoperative pain, often providing better control of pain than systemic opioids.

**Sympathetic** nerves are part of the autonomic nervous system. Sympathetic nerves are found in both the central nervous system (CNS) (preganglionic) and the peripheral nervous system (postganglionic). Those in the CNS communicate with those in the peripheral system through a series of ganglia by means of neurotransmitters (acetylcholine) at synapses. The sympathetic nervous system (T1-L2 or L3) is activated in times of stress and is implicated in pain. The nerves innervate deep structures, viscera, and skin. Ganglia are paired: 3 cervical, 12 thoracic, 4 lumbar, 4 sacral, and 1 impar (at the coccyx). Sympathetic blocks (subarachnoid, epidural, paravertebral) provide pain relief for visceral pain, herpetic neuralgia, postherpetic pain, and peripheral vascular disease.

## Somatic nerve blocks (trigeminal)

Somatic nerve blocks include **trigeminal nerve blocks**, most commonly used for severe facial cancer pain and performed on the gasserian ganglion or its branches:

- *Gasserian ganglion block:* This block requires an anterolateral approach under radiographic guidance with insertion 3 cm lateral to the mouth angle (at the level of the second upper molar).
- *Ophthalmic nerve block:* Usually only the supraoptic branch is blocked so that keratitis can be avoided. Insertion is at the supraoptic ridge superior to the pupil. The supratrochlear branch may also be blocked.
- *Maxillary nerve block:* This block affects the maxillary nerve along with the pterygopalatine ganglia, with insertion between the zygomatic arch and the mandible notch. The needle is angled anteriorly.
- *Mandibular nerve block:* The insertion point is for the maxillary nerve, but the needle is directed posteriorly toward the ear.
- *Supraorbital nerve block:* The insertion point is at the supraorbital notch.

## Somatic nerve blocks (intercostal)

**Somatic nerve blocks** to control chest and upper abdominal pain include the following:

- *Intercostal block*: These nerves arise from the thoracic spinal nerves, running along a groove on the posterior surface of each rib along with the arteries and veins, and innervating the skin and muscles of the chest and abdomen. This block is used for analgesia after rib fractures and surgery of the chest (mastectomy, thoracotomy) or upper abdomen (gastrostomy, cholecystectomy), although it is not effective for visceral pain. The block requires the patient to be seated, lying prone, or in the lateral decubitus position; insertion is at the proximal to the midaxillary line, inferior to the rib, often at the rib angle. Most blocks are at T7 or lower. Intercostal blocks result in the highest blood levels of anesthetic agents; therefore, the patient must be monitored carefully for indications of toxicity. Pneumothorax can occur easily if the needle is misdirected. Although this block is a good adjunct for pain, patients almost always also require systemic medications.

## Somatic nerve blocks (facial, glossopharyngeal, occipital)

**Somatic nerve blocks** of the neck, face, and head are used to control various types of pain:

- *Facial nerve block:* This block may be administered to relieve the pain of herpes zoster (affecting this nerve) or spastic facial contractions. The insertion point is anterior to the mastoid process, inferior to the mandibular ramus (1-2 cm deep). Injection too deep may result in a block of the glossopharyngeal or vagus nerves.
- *Glossopharyngeal block:* This block is effective for control of mouth pain, such as that caused by malignancies of the base of the tongue, the epiglottis, or the palatine tonsils. It may also be used to distinguish glossopharyngeal neuralgia from other types (such as trigeminal). Dysphagia and ipsilateral vocal cord paralysis may result from the block.
- *Occipital block:* This block may be used to treat and diagnose occipital headaches. The occipital nerve is accessed 3 cm lateral to the occipital prominence at the superior nuchal line.

## Somatic blocks (paravertebral)

**Paravertebral somatic blocks** involve injection of anesthetic agent approximately 2.5 cm lateral to the spinous process of the target vertebra or nerve, a space lateral to point at which the nerve leaves the intervertebral foramina. Paravertebral blocks are used to control of unilateral acute and chronic pain:

- *Cervical block*: This block is used at C2-C7. Insertion is often performed under fluoroscopic guidance to avoid intravascular, intrathecal, subdural, or epidural placement, which may result in severe respiratory compromise, seizures, or both. This block is particularly useful for patients with cancer pain related to the cervical spine or shoulder.
- *Thoracic block*: This block provides analgesia at a higher level than the intercostal block and is used for pain from the thoracic spine, thoracic rib cage, and abdominal wall, including herpes and fractures. Because pneumothorax is the most common complication, chest radiography should be performed after the block.
- *Lumbar block*: This block is used for evaluation of pain related to the lumbar spine. Most complications relate to incorrect injection (intravascular, intrathecal, subdural, or epidural).

## Somatic blocks (diaphragm and shoulder)

**Somatic blocks** may be used to relive pain in the diaphragm and shoulder:

- *Phrenic block:* The phrenic nerve arises at C3-C5 and innervates the central diaphragm; therefore, this block may relief pain in that origin or refractory hiccups. The insertion point is 3 cm superior to the clavicle, lateral to the posterior border of the sternocleidomastoid muscle and above the anterior scalene muscle. This block may cause respiratory compromise in patients with preexisting pulmonary disease and should never be given bilaterally.
- *Suprascapular block:* The suprascapular nerve is the primary nerve providing sensation to the shoulder joint, but it also provides motor function to the supraspinatus and infraspinatus muscles. The nerve arises from the brachial plexus at the level of C4-C6. The insertion point is at the supraspinal notch, using care to avoid pneumothorax. Motor paralysis of the supraspinatus and infraspinatus is one complication. This block is most commonly used to relieve joint pain related to arthritis or bursitis.

### Somatic nerve blocks (transsacral and pudendal)

**Somatic nerve blocks** may be used to control intractable pain in the pelvic and perineal area:

- **Transsacral block:** This block is especially useful for pelvic or perineal pain, especially pain related to cancer, such as bladder cancer, and sometimes lower back pain. One or more blocks of the sacral nerves may be performed, depending on the location and degree of pain. Injections are given bilaterally because the nerves are paired (5 paired sacral nerves and 1 pair of coccygeal nerves). Injection is into the posterior sacral foramen.
- *Pudendal:* The pudendal nerve, arising from S2-S4, may be blocked to treat (as during delivery) or evaluate perineal pain. The injection site is posterior to the ischial spine at the sacrospinous ligament attachment (palpated transvaginally or transrectally). Care must be taken to avoid sciatic blockade. This block is often performed bilaterally but may not always provide adequate bilateral analgesia. This block is performed with the patient in the lithotomy position.

### Sympathetic blocks (stellate)

**Sympathetic blocks** that selectively block only sympathetic nerve fibers are useful in determining the degree to which the sympathetic system contributes to pain. An isolated sympathetic block should not alter somatic sensation and should increase both blood flow and tissue temperature:

- *Stellate (cervicothoracic) block:* The inferior cervical ganglion and the T1 ganglion fuse to form the stellate ganglion at C7. Block of the stellate ganglion may relieve pain in the head, neck, arm, and upper chest, and may block to the T5 level, depending on the amount of anesthetic agent. Injection is made with the patient supine and the neck extended. The needle is usually inserted at the C6 level (because insertion at the C7 level is more likely to result in pneumothorax) between the trachea and the carotid sheath. Aspiration and test doses are used to ensure that there is no intravascular injection, because arteries (vertebral and subclavian) are in close proximity.

### Sympathetic blocks (lumbar and hypogastric)

**Sympathetic blocks** may be used to treat pain in the pelvis and lower extremities:

- *Lumbar block:* The lumbar sympathetic chain contains 3 to 5 ganglia. This block is frequently used to reduce pain and swelling in the lower extremities and to improve mobility. It is specifically used for pelvic pain, herpes zoster, reflex sympathetic dystrophy, peripheral vascular disease, and complex regional pain syndrome. Injection is usually performed under fluoroscopic guidance with a 2-needle technique at L2 and L4. A series of injections may be given, sometimes weekly, until the pain subsides. Transient weakness and numbness of the legs may occur after the block.
- *Hypogastric block:* The hypogastric plexus contains visceral sensory nerve fibers from the cervix, uterus, bladder, prostate, and rectum. The superior hypogastric plexus is at L5, and the inferior plexus is at S2-S4. This block is used for pelvic pain that is unresponsive to lumbar or caudal epidurals; it is most commonly used for patients with cancer or nonmalignant pain of these organs. The insertion point is 7 cm lateral to the L4-L5 spinal interspace.

### Sympathetic blocks (celiac plexus)

**Sympathetic nerve blocks** may be used to treat abdominal visceral pain:

- *Celiac plexus block:* The celiac plexus lies behind the peritoneum in the upper abdomen at T12 and L1 and is a network of both sympathetic and parasympathetic nerves with 2 ganglia receiving sympathetic nerves. It provides nerves for the gastrointestinal system (including stomach, intestines, gallbladder, liver, and pancreas) and for the kidneys and adrenal glands. Celiac plexus block is used to block visceral pain, especially pain related to malignancies. Injection may be performed on the left or bilaterally, often with guidance provided by CT or fluoroscopy. Insertion is at L1, 3 to 8 cm from the midline of the inferior edge of the spinous process. This site is often used for neurolytic blocks with 50% to 100% alcohol, along with an anesthetic agent to reduce the pain of alcohol injection. Complications include postural hypotension. Severe systemic reactions can occur with inadvertent intravascular injection into the vena cava.

### Intrathecal (spinal) narcotics

Intrathecal (subarachnoid or spinal) administration of opioids is used for patients whose pain is not controlled by other methods (such as oral, IM, or IV drugs). **Intrathecal narcotics** (commonly morphine, fentanyl, or a combination) are frequently administered during surgical procedures employing a spinal anesthetic or as an adjunct to general anesthesia to control postoperative pain. Opioids bind with receptors at the dorsal horn to block pain signals. If morphine is used, analgesia begins within 20 to 60 minutes and lasts for 12 to 36 hours, but this effect is dose-dependent. Pruritus is a common adverse effect (40%). Intrathecal administration during surgery tends to reduce postsurgical pain, even after the effect wanes. Intrathecal catheters may be implanted or placed percutaneously for continuous use. An indwelling device may be placed in the right lower quadrant of the abdomen with an intrathecal pump to control administration and a tunneling catheter from the lumbosacral area. Intrathecal analgesia is somewhat less predictable than epidural; adverse effects, such as respiratory depression, may be delayed but may result from excessive dosage.

### Patient-controlled analgesia

**Patient-controlled analgesia** (PCA) allows the patient to control the administration of pain medication by pressing a button on an intravenous delivery system with a computerized pump. The device is filled with opioid (as prescribed) and must be programmed correctly and checked regularly to ensure that it is functioning properly and that controls are set. The most commonly administered medications include morphine, meperidine, fentanyl, and sufentanil. Most devices can be set to deliver a continuous infusion of opioid as well as a patient-controlled bolus. Each element must be set:

- *Bolus*: Determines the amount of medication received when the patient delivers a dose.
- *Lockout interval:* Time required between administration of boluses.
- *Continuous infusion:* Rate at which opioid is delivered per hour for continuous analgesia.
- *Limit* (usually set at 4 hours): Total amount of opioid that can be delivered within the preset time limit.

After knee procedures specifically, it has been shown that having a continuous infusion is just as effective at controlling pain as an epidural infusion. With Authorized Agent Controlled Analgesia

(AACA), persons who are trained and authorized (such as nurse, family member, and caregiver) may also administer the medication to the patient.

# Other Techniques

### Spinal anesthesia

Patients receiving spinal anesthesia are particularly sensitive to sedative medications and prone to oversedation. These patients are more likely to experience respiratory and cardiac arrest after receiving sedatives. This arrest tends to be very difficult to resuscitate and results in high morbidity, and in those who survive, high incidence of neurological deficit.

Total spinal anesthesia can result when there is depression of the cervical spinal cord and the brainstem after having local spinal anesthesia. Patients have symptoms including loss of consciousness, hypotension, bradycardia, and cardiac arrest. The patient should have their airway immediately secured and mechanical ventilation initiated. The injury results in a loss of sympathetic tone, so their management during arrest, in addition to typical ACLS protocol, will include escalating the dose of epinephrine. This patient would receive 1mg epinephrine, then 2mg, then 4mg, etc.

### Hypothermia during anesthesia

**Hypothermia** (<36°C) often occurs intentionally or unintentionally during surgery. Core temperatures decrease during surgery, and the body cannot compensate because of anesthetic-induced thermoregulatory impairment. A number of steps are used to prevent hypothermia: prewarming with forced-air or other types of warming blankets (this has been proven to be the best way to rewarm the patient as well), heating of IV fluids, increasing ambient room temperature, and heated humidifiers. However, in some types of surgery (craniotomy, cardiac surgery), intentional hypothermia is induced by the use of a cooling blanket to decrease oxygen requirements and slow metabolism as a protective method for the heart and brain. Cooling blankets are usually placed beneath and over the patient and are set at approximately 5°C until the target core temperature has been reached. Temperature is usually monitored with an esophageal probe. Deep hypothermia (15-22°C) risks more complications than more moderate hypothermia (32-34°C). The patient is rewarmed at the end of the procedure, beginning in the operating room and continuing into the recovery area, until the body temperature reaches a target normal rate.

### Controlled hypotension during surgery

**Controlled hypotension** may be used for some surgical procedures (cerebral aneurysm, brain tumor, total hip arthroplasty, radical neck resection) to minimize blood loss during the procedure and improve visualization. Blood pressure lowering is usually achieved by some combination of patient positioning (elevating the surgical site), hypotensive drugs, and positive-pressure ventilation to decrease cardiac output, venous return, and arterial blood pressure. A high sympathetic block (epidural or subarachnoid) may also produce hypotension. Controlled hypotension is contraindicated for patients with severe anemia, hypovolemia, or other conditions that may prevent adequate perfusion of organs. The level of controlled hypotension that can be achieved varies. A mean arterial pressure of 50 to 60 mm Hg may be safe for younger patients, but patients with some hypertension may tolerate only a 20% to 30% reduction. Careful monitoring of intraarterial blood pressure and ECG is necessary throughout the surgical procedure.

# Postanesthesia Care/Respiratory Care

## Standards of postanesthesia care

The **American Society of PeriAnesthesia Nurses** (ASPAN) has delineated standards (modified in 2004) for postanesthesia management of patients. There are 5 standards:

1. Patients must receive management of care in an appropriate postanesthesia care unit (PACU) according to accreditation and licensing requirements.
2. The patient must be accompanied to the unit by a knowledgeable member of the anesthesia team, and the patient must be continually monitored during transport.
3. A complete report (including preoperative and operative information) must be provided to the staff receiving the patient in the postanesthesia unit, and the member of the anesthesia team must stay in the unit until the staff accepts responsibility for the patient.
4. The patient must be continually monitored (oxygenation, level of consciousness, temperature, circulation, ventilation), and findings must be documented. A physician must be available to manage complications.
5. A physician must be responsible for discharging the patient from the unit, or preestablished discharge criteria must be met.

## Emergence from anesthesia

**Emergence** from anesthesia must be carefully managed and will vary depending on the type of anesthetic agents used. If muscle relaxants are used to paralyze muscles during surgery, then the effects must be reversed before emergence and removal of ventilation so that the patient can breathe independently. Administration of the muscle relaxant is discontinued, and a reversing agent, such as an anticholinesterase, may be used. With general anesthesia, patients may be able to follow verbal directions soon after the anesthetic agent has been discontinued and the intubation tube can be removed, unless the patient is to be continued on ventilation. In that case, the patient may be transferred to the postanesthesia unit before awakening. Patients may have some persistent difficulty with thinking after emergence because of the lasting effects of some anesthetic agents. Because of respiratory depression, a common adverse effect of most anesthetic agents, careful monitoring of oxygen saturation and ventilation is required during the recovery period, and supplemental oxygen is provided to improve oxygen saturation.

## Postoperative nausea and vomiting (PONV)

**Postoperative nausea and vomiting** (PONV) varies with the type of anesthetic agent used. It occurs in approximately 20% to 30% of postanesthesia patients and may be delayed for as long as 24 hours. Inhalational agents are associated with a higher incidence of PONV than intravenous agents, and the incidence is lower with epidural or subarachnoid administration, although it may indicate the onset of hypotension. PONV correlates with the duration of the surgical procedure: longer procedures cause increased PONV. If high doses of narcotics, propofol, or nitrous oxide are used, PONV is often a problem. PONV is most common among young women and also relates to menstruation. It is also more likely among patients with a history of smoking or motion sickness. Some surgical procedures are more likely to be associated with PONV: strabismus repair, ear surgery, laparoscopy, tonsillectomy, orchiopexy, and gynecological procedures for retrieving ova. PONV may be associated with postoperative pain; therefore, managing pain is an important factor in preventing PONV.

### Delayed emergence

**Delayed emergence** (failure to emerge for 30 to 60 minutes after anesthesia ends) is more common in the elderly because of slowed metabolism of anesthetic agents, but it may have a variety of causes, such as drug overdose during surgery or overdose related to preinduction use of drugs or alcohol that potentiates intraoperative drugs. In this case, naloxone or flumazenil may be indicated if opioids or benzodiazepines are implicated. Physostigmine may also be used to reverse the effects of some anesthetic agents. Hypothermia may also cause a delay in emergence, especially core temperatures are lower than 33°C, and forced-air warming blankets may be required for increasing the temperature. Other metabolic conditions, such as hypoglycemia or hyperglycemia, may also affect emergence. Patients experiencing delayed emergence must be evaluated for perioperative stroke, especially after neurological, cardiovascular, or cerebrovascular surgery. Metabolic disturbance may also delay emergence.

### Respiratory complications

**Respiratory complications** are the most common during the postanesthesia period; therefore, monitoring of oxygen levels is crucial for preventing hypoxemia:

- *Airway obstruction* may be partial or total. Partial obstruction is indicated by sonorous or wheezing respirations, and total obstruction by absence of breath sounds. Treatment includes supplemental oxygen, airway insertion, repositioning (jaw thrust), or succinylcholine and positive-pressure ventilation for laryngospasm. If edema of the glottis is causing obstruction, IV corticosteroids may be used.
- *Hypoventilation* ($Paco_2$ >45 mm Hg) is often mild but may cause respiratory acidosis. It is usually related to depression caused by anesthetic agents. A number of factors may slow emergence (hypothermia, overdose, metabolism) and cause hypoventilation. It may also be related to splinting because of pain, requiring additional pain management.
- *Hypoxemia* (mild, $Pao_2$ 50 to 60 mm Hg) is usually related to hypoventilation, increased right-to-left shunting, or both and is usually treated with supplementary oxygen (30% to 60%) with or without positive airway pressure.

### Cardiovascular complications

**Cardiovascular complications** are sometimes related to respiratory complications, which may also need to be addressed. Complications include the following:

- *Hypotension* is most often mild and requires no specific treatment. It is most commonly caused by hypovolemia and is significant if BP falls to 20% to 30% below normal baseline. A bolus (100-250 mL IV colloid) is used to confirm hypovolemia. If hypotension is severe, medications, such as epinephrine, may be indicated. Because hypotension may occur with pneumothorax, careful respiratory assessment is necessary.
- *Hypertension* usually occurs no more than 30 minutes after surgery and is common among patients with a history of hypertension. It may be secondary to hypoxemia or metabolic acidosis. Mild increases in BP usually do not require treatment, but medications may be used for moderate (β-adrenergic blockers) or severe (nitroprusside) hypertension.
- *Arrhythmias* usually relate to respiratory complications or the effects of anesthetic agents. Bradycardia may relate to cholinesterase inhibitors, opioids, or propranolol. Tachycardia may relate to anticholinergics, β-agonists, and vagolytic drugs. Hypokalemia and hypomagnesemia may cause premature atrial and ventricular beats.

# Pain Theory

## Types of pain (nociceptive)

There are two **primary types of pain**: nociceptive (acute) pain and neuropathic pain, although some people may have a combination:

- **Nociceptive** or acute pain is the normal nerve response to a painful stimulus. Trauma that results in nociceptive pain can cause severe inflammation and damage to nerve endings. Nociceptive pain usually correlates with extent and type of injury: the more severe the injury, the greater the pain. It may be procedural pain (related to wound manipulation and dressing changes) or surgical pain (related to cutting of tissue). It may also be continuous or cyclic, depending on the type of injury. This type of pain is usually localized to the area of injury and resolves over time as healing takes place. This type of pain is often described as aching or throbbing, but it generally responds to analgesia. It has been shown that effective pain control can decrease complications in the postoperative period. Uncontrolled, this type of pain can in time result in changes in the nervous system that lead to chronic neuropathic pain.
- **Neuropathic pain** occurs when there is a primary lesion in the nervous system or dysfunction related to damaged nerve fibers. Often the underlying pathology causing the pain is not reversible. It is often diffused rather than localized. It may also be somatic pain (involving muscles, skin, bones, and joints). Neuropathic pain is often more difficult to assess than nociceptive pain because the damage may alter normal pain responses. Neuropathic pain often responds better to antidepressants and antiseizure medications than to analgesics, and addressing underlying psychologic conditions can help with recovery. This type of pain most effectively treated using a holistic approach to include psychological support, physical and occupational therapy, medication, nerve blocks and implantable devices.

After undergoing a new surgery, patients who have chronic neuropathic pain will usually need triple the normal dose of opioids for two days. Peripheral nerve blocks often benefit these patients as well. This patient population will often benefit from an analgesic adjunct like gabapentin or a COX-2 inhibitor like celecoxib (usually only taken for 5 days max).

## Averse systemic effects of pain

Acute pain causes **adverse systemic affects** that can negatively affect many body systems Pain is now considered the fifth vital sign, and it should be assessed using objective scales and ability to perform ADLs and other daily functions.

- ***Cardiovascular***: Tachycardia and increased BP is a common response to pain, causing increased cardiac output and systemic vascular resistance. In patients with preexisting cardiovascular disease, such as compromised ventricular function, cardiac output may decrease. The increased myocardial need for oxygen may cause or worsen myocardial ischemia.
- ***Respiratory***: Increased need for oxygen causes an increase in minute ventilation, and splinting because of pain may compromise pulmonary function. If the chest wall movement is constrained, tidal volume falls, impairing the ability to cough and clear secretions. Bed rest further compromises ventilation.

- *Gastrointestinal*: Sphincter tone increases and motility decreases, sometimes resulting in ileus. There may be increased secretion of gastric acids, which irritate the gastric lining and can cause ulcerations. Nausea, vomiting, and constipation may occur. Reflux may result in aspiration pneumonia. Abdominal distention may occur.
- *Urinary*: Increased sphincter tone and decreased motility result in urinary retention.
- *Endocrine*: Hormone levels are affected by pain. The levels of catabolic hormones, such as catecholamine, cortisol, and glucagon, increase; the levels of anabolic hormones, such as insulin and testosterone, decrease. Lipolysis increases along with carbohydrate intolerance. Sodium retention can occur because of increased ADH, aldosterone, angiotensin, and cortisol. This in turn causes fluid retention and a shift to the extracellular space.
- *Hematologic*: There may be reduced fibrinolysis, increased adhesiveness of platelets, and increased coagulation.
- *Immune*: Leukocytosis and lymphopenia may occur, increasing the risk of infection.
- *Emotional*: Patients may become depressed, anxious, or angry; may have a depressed appetite; and may be sleep-deprived. This type of response is most common among those with chronic pain, who usually do not have systemic responses typical of patients with acute pain.

## Chronic neuropathic pain

There are many types of **chronic pain** (back pain, migraines, herpetic), and most are treated without anesthetic agents. Chronic low back pain (persisting for more than 3 months) can be severely debilitating, and its control may require multidimensional approaches (NSAIDs, physiotherapy, antidepressants). If pain has persisted for more than 6 months, intradiscal electrothermal therapy (IDET), in which a special probe is inserted into the disk and heated, may shrink the disk and relieve pain. Neuropathic pain may result from a number of conditions, such as diabetic neuropathy, postherpetic neuralgia, and stroke. Pain may be burning, hyperpathic, and paroxysmal. Many approaches to pain control may be necessary, including NSAIDs, tricyclic antidepressants (amitriptyline), and anticonvulsants (gabapentin). In some cases, patients respond well to sympathetic blocks that targeting the nerves that trigger pain, if the blocks are given in conjunction with adjuvant treatments. In other cases, such as herpes zoster, a sympathetic block during the acute stage may reduce chronic pain, but the block is generally ineffective if given after the pain has become chronic.

# Advanced Principles of Anesthesia

## Surgical Procedures and Procedures related to Organ Systems

### Gall bladder removal (cholecystectomy)

Acute **gall bladder** disease is usually stabilized before surgery, except for acalculous cholecystitis or severe cholangitis, which may require emergency surgery. ***Cholecystectomy*** is usually performed laparoscopically with insufflation of carbon dioxide into the abdomen, which increases abdominal pressure. Additionally, the Trendelenburg position may be used to shift abdominal organs away from the operative site. These techniques combine to decrease ventilation and venous return; therefore, adequate IV fluids and respiratory monitoring are essential. End-tidal $CO_2$ concentrations are monitored because some systemic absorption of $CO_2$ can occur. If an intraoperative cholangiogram is performed, opioid administration may be limited because opioids can cause spasm of the sphincter of Oddi. Drugs that are dependent on biliary excretion should be avoided in the presence of biliary tract obstruction in favor of those that are dependent on renal excretion. Decompressing the stomach with an NG tube may prevent inadvertent puncture when the needle is inserted for insufflation. Nitrous oxide is usually avoided because it could expand gases in the intestines.

### Liver disease and surgery

**Liver disease** affects all body systems. Cirrhosis of the liver combined with anesthesia-induced hypotension and decreased cardiac output may cause ischemia of the liver. Additionally, hepatic blood flow may be impaired by positive-pressure pulmonary ventilation, congestive heart failure, and excess fluids. The degree of decrease in blood flow correlates with the proximity of the surgical site to the liver. The stress of surgery may cause hyperglycemia as glycogen breakdown accelerates. Liver disease may also contribute to coagulopathy, which may be treated with the administration of red blood cells, fresh frozen plasma (FFP), platelets, or medications, such as conjugated estrogen or activated recombinant factor VII. Liver disease may limit the use of anesthetic agents metabolized in the liver. For example, elimination half-times may be prolonged with certain drugs (morphine, alfentanil, and diazepam). CNS depressant may be avoided with end-stage liver disease. With intact cardiac and respiratory function, induction is with IV anesthetic, opioids, and NMBAs. Rapid-sequence anesthesia should be used with ascites. Vasoconstrictors may be used to combat hypotension. Inhalation anesthetic gases can cause toxicity leading to hepatic dysfunction, with halothane being the most often implicated of the gases (though rarely used in the U.S.). As all the inhalation gases cause hepatic artery and preportal blood vessel, they lead to portal flow decrease. Subsequently, patients with liver disease should be anesthesized at levels below 1 MAC.

### Pancreas

The **pancreas** contains both exocrine tissue (producing digestive enzymes) and endocrine tissue (producing hormones, such as insulin). Therefore, pancreatic surgery, which interferes with pancreatic function, can cause a number of complications. Surgery may be necessary for removal of tumors, incision and drainage, acute pancreatitis, and transplantation. An abdominal incision or a laparoscopic approach is used, and postoperative drains are inserted during the procedure. Anesthesia may be inhalational (sometimes with epidural infusion) or intravenous. Hypotension is treated with adequate IV fluids and sometimes vasopressors. Patients who are diabetic pose many problems, including a high rate (30%) of difficult airways. Diabetic patients often have coronary artery disease, hypertension, and neuropathy that must be managed during surgery. A continuous

- 23 -

insulin infusion may be indicated for controlling glucose levels. The formula for insulin administration is used to maintain serum glucose at 120 to 180 mg/dL:

- Regular insulin units = serum glucose level (mg/dL) divided by 150 (or 100 for patients receiving corticosteroids that equal 100 mg prednisone daily).

Postoperative pain may be managed by a thoracic epidural infusion, PCA, or both.

### Spleen

The **spleen** is a small bean-shaped organ in the upper left abdomen. It serves as a reservoir for approximately 30% of platelets, filters the blood, and controls blood flow to the liver. Splenectomy (complete or partial) may be preformed for hypersplenism, trauma, cancer, hereditary spherocytosis, and immune thrombocytopenic purpura (ITP). Surgery is conducted with the patient under general anesthesia with an abdominal incision or with laparoscopy (unless splenomegaly is pronounced). If the spleen is enlarged, the artery to the spleen is tied before the ligaments are loosened and the organ is removed. If the organ has ruptured, the splenic artery is tied from underneath and the organ is then removed. Preoperatively, blood loss or coagulopathy must be treated. Postoperatively, the patient is at increased risk of infection and sepsis, and children may receive antibiotic prophylaxis until they reach the age of 16. Adults may also receive penicillin for 2 years or ampicillin for long-term prophylaxis. Preoperative vaccinations are given for elective procedures.

### Stomach (gastrectomy) surgical procedures

**Gastrectomy** with removal of all or part of the stomach may be used to treat GI hemorrhage, gastric cancer, gastric perforation, or polyps. Gastrectomy generally requires insertion of a nasogastric tube for irrigation and decompression of the stomach. In emergency procedures for gastric hemorrhage, the patient is at increased risk of respiratory compromise due to aspiration of blood or gastric fluids; immediate intubation and ventilation may be necessary for protecting the airway. Additionally, hypovolemia and electrolyte imbalances must be managed before induction. Balanced anesthesia (intravenous and inhalational anesthetics) is often used and is sometimes combined with thoracic epidural. Surgery is usually performed with an abdominal incision, but laparoscopy may be possible in some cases. After all or part of the stomach has been removed, the small intestine is attached to the esophagus (for total gastrectomy) or to the remaining stomach (for partial gastrectomy). Epidural infusion may be used for postoperative pain management.

### Renal

Approximately 20% to 25% of the cardiac output each minute is filtered through the **kidney**, with a renal blood flow (RBF) of approximately 1200 mL/min and a glomerular filtration rate (GFR) of 125 mL/min. The stress created by surgery and anesthesia on the body's systems can decrease both the RBF and the GFR, resulting in decrease in water and sodium excretion (more pronounced with general than with regional anesthesia). These changes often relate to hypovolemia and are reversible with fluid administration.

The preferred muscle relaxant in patients with renal diasease is atracurium, although succinylcholine may be used if hyperkalemia is not present. Though dopamine has been used in the past for its alleged renoprotective properties, there is now evidence that dopamine does not improve renal perfusion. Spinal and epidural anesthesia depress kidney function, but this is reversible. General anesthesia depresses kidney function to an even greater degree than spinal or epidural, but as with the later two, it is reversible and most effects can be minimized by obtaining preoperative euvolemia and blood pressure control.

The anesthetics used during intraabdominal surgery may have a direct effect on the kidneys. Some anesthetic agents are toxic to the kidneys in high doses (methoxyflurane, enflurane, sevoflurane) and may result in renal failure. Other agents (halothane, enflurane, and isoflurane) decrease renal vascular resistance. Enflurane may cause increased plasma fluoride concentrations in the obese or those on isoniazid (INH) therapy. Intravenous agents, such as opioids and barbiturates, when combined with nitrous oxide may cause effects similar to those of volatile anesthetics. Many other drugs prevent the kidneys from adapting to changes during anesthesia and result in decreased GFR. Preexisting renal disease exacerbates reactions to drugs, such as antibiotics, immunosuppressive drugs, and contrast dyes. Acetylcysteine may provide protection against contrast dye-induced renal failure. Surgical procedures themselves may interfere with renal function. Laparoscopic procedures induce a pneumoperitoneum with increased intraabdominal pressure that decreases urinary output. Cardiovascular surgery, especially with cardiopulmonary bypass, may impair renal function.

## Radical nephrectomy

**Radical nephrectomy** is done for adenocarcinoma of the kidney, which may be associated with paraneoplastic syndromes. Because this type of cancer is associated with smoking, patients may have underlying coronary artery or respiratory disease. Some patients have erythrocytosis, but many are anemic and may require transfusions in preparation for surgery to increase hemoglobin to at least 10 g/dL. Surgery is performed with the patient under endotracheal general anesthesia with an anterior subcostal, flank, or thoracoabdominal (preferred for large tumors) incision. The kidney and its adrenal gland with surrounding fat and fascia are removed together. Blood loss may be extensive because the tumors tend to be vascular and large, requiring multiple transfusions. However, controlled hypotension should be limited to brief periods because it may impair renal function. Mannitol is given before dissection. Continual direct arterial pressure monitoring and central venous cannulation are necessary.

## Radical nephrectomy with tumor thrombus

In some cases of **radical nephrectomy,** a **tumor thrombus** extends from the kidney into the inferior vena cava. This condition complicates anesthesia, because invasive monitoring is necessary. The thrombus may extend below the liver (level I), below the diaphragm (level II), or into the right atrium (level III). Multiple intravenous catheters must be in place because blood loss may be extensive with tumor thrombus, sometimes requiring the administration of more than 50 units of packed cells. Platelets, fresh frozen plasma (FFP), and cryoprecipitate are usually given. If the thrombus obstructs the vena cava, patients are at increased risk of bleeding and pulmonary embolization of the tumor, which are often associated with pronounced hypotension, supraventricular arrhythmias, and oxygen desaturation. Heparinization and hypothermia may be used, but they increase blood loss. Cardiopulmonary bypass may be used if the tumor extends into the right atrium, occupying more than 40% of the atrium. In cases in which the tumor extends into the vena cava, the purpose of surgery is not curative rather to prolong and improve the quality of life.

## Diaphragm

The **diaphragm** is the musculomembranous partition separating the abdominal and thoracic cavities; it is innervated by the phrenic nerve, which arises from C3 to C5. Abdominal and thoracic

- 25 -

surgical procedures with the patient under general anesthesia (combined IV and inhalation) can compromise the function of the diaphragm, resulting a decrease of approximately 20% in functional residual capacity. Additionally, irritation of the phrenic nerve may decrease contractility of the diaphragmatic muscles. Epidural thoracic anesthesia is less disruptive of the diaphragm than general anesthesia, causing fewer pulmonary adverse effects (such as hypoxemia and atelectasis). Nitrous oxide is usually avoided in surgical repairs of the diaphragm itself because it may lead to an increase in intraabdominal pressure that may result in ischemia. Thoracic or abdominal surgery, such as open-heart surgery, can result in unilateral or bilateral paralysis of the diaphragm, causing accessory muscles to attempt to compensate. Patients with unilateral paralysis may exhibit few symptoms at rest but exhibit dyspnea with exertion. Bilateral paralysis causes profound respiratory distress; total lung capacity often decreases by 50%, necessitating mechanical ventilation.

## Intestines (loop ileostomy/colostomy)

A **loop ileostomy** may be a temporary fecal diversion or an alternative to a double lumen colostomy to allow healing distally for conditions such as rectovaginal fistula. The procedure is usually performed with the patient under general anesthesia with either a midline abdominal incision or with laparoscopy with a small incision in the lower right abdomen. The patient is usually supine in pronounced Trendelenburg position of at least 40° to shift the viscera and intestines toward the thoracic cavity. The patient is secured with cushioning under the knees and lower legs and with the right arm extended for anesthesia access. A loop of the small intestine is brought through the abdominal wall, positioned, and incised; the afferent loop is everted and sutured to create a cone-like stoma, and the efferent loop is sutured flat to the abdomen. The **double-lumen colostomy** is performed with similar surgical procedures on the sigmoid colon, pulling a loop through the abdominal wall with a spacer bar beneath the loop, incising, and suturing an active stoma and a terminal stoma.

## Herniorrhaphy

**Hernia repair (herniorrhaphy)** is the most common surgical procedure for infants and children and is also common for adults. Surgery is performed to repair herniation of the peritoneum with a segment of bowel through the abdominal wall to prevent an incarcerated hernia. There are 3 main types:

- *Inguinal:* Herniation in the inguinal canal. This is common in premature or low birth weight infants, usually boys, and may occur bilaterally. It is also common in men.
- *Femoral:* Herniation posterior to the inguinal ligament. This is more common in female patients.
- *Umbilical:* Herniation in the umbilical ring.

Inguinal and femoral hernias are usually repaired early because of the danger of incarceration; however, umbilical hernias in children often heal over time without surgical repair. If incarceration has occurred before surgery, the affected segment of bowel is resected. Surgery may be performed laparoscopically. General anesthesia is the most common, but subarachnoid or local infiltration anesthesia is effective and often decreases postoperative recovery time.

## Bladder (radical cystectomy)

**Radical cystectomy** is performed for bladder cancer (most commonly transitional cell carcinoma) and also involves removal of the prostate and seminal vesicles of male patients and removal of the uterus, cervix, ovaries, and a portion of the anterior vaginal vault of female patients. A urinary diversion is created after removal of the bladder. Radical cystectomy is an extensive operation, requiring 4 to 6 hours of general endotracheal anesthesia combined with a muscle relaxant. The patient is placed in the hyperextended supine position. Controlled hypotension may be used to reduce bleeding and improve visualization, and this may be facilitated by the concurrent use of spinal or epidural anesthesia with general anesthesia, although neuraxial anesthesia may cause hyperperistalsis of the bowel, complicating construction of a reservoir for urinary diversion. Blood loss may be extensive; therefore, close monitoring of blood pressure, blood loss, and intravascular pressure is necessary because blood transfusions may be required. Urinary output must be monitored continually. A forced-air warming blanket is placed over the upper body so that hypothermia can be prevented.

## Ovarian cyst

**Ovarian cysts** are usually benign functional cysts that may recede without surgical intervention, but if they cause pain or symptoms or if the woman is menopausal and older than 50, the cyst may be removed via laparotomy with the patient under general anesthesia or via laparoscopy with the patient under local or general (most common) anesthesia. Laparoscopy allows for visualization of the pelvic area, washing for cytologic examination, and biopsy (in some cases). If the cyst is to be removed, either the entire ovary or a part of it will be removed. In many cases, an attempt is made to remove only the cyst, keeping the walls intact. The cyst is sometimes placed in a plastic sack before removal to ensure that it remains intact. Dermoid cysts, especially, must be handled with care because they contain various tissue types, and if these cysts leak, they can cause severe adhesions or peritonitis. In case of leakage, the area is lavaged. If the ovary is severely damaged or if there is a familial history of ovarian cancer, the entire ovary may be removed.

## Prostatectomy (radical retropubic)

**Radical retropubic prostatectomy** is performed for prostate cancer (adenocarcinoma) with the patient under general endotracheal anesthesia with a lower midline abdominal incision and the patient in the hyperextended supine position. Surgery includes pelvic lymph node dissection. The seminal vesicles, ejaculatory ducts, and part of the bladder neck are removed, and the urethra is reattached at the remaining bladder neck. Blood loss is often substantial; therefore, direct arterial pressure and central venous pressure (CVP) should be monitored. Controlled hypotension may be used to reduce blood loss. The procedure may be performed with the patient under neuraxial anesthesia (T6 sensory level), but heavy sedation is required because of the discomfort associated with the positioning, and edema of the airway can occur because of the position coupled with intravenous fluids. A laparoscopic prostatectomy may be possible, but the steep Trendelenburg (>30°) position increases the chance of $CO_2$ absorption from the retroperitoneum; therefore, careful $CO_2$ monitoring is necessary. Nitrous oxide is usually avoided with $CO_2$ insufflation.

## Laparoscopy

**Laparoscopy** is a minimally invasive procedure increasingly used for abdominal surgery. The patient is anesthetized and placed in the Trendelenburg position. Laparoscopy involves one or more small incisions. An incision 0.5 to 2 cm long is used for the trochar and laparoscope, but smaller ports (incisions) may be used for instruments that assist with the operative procedure. Laparoscopy is associated with less dysfunction of the diaphragm and faster recovery because of smaller incisions and less manipulation. Laparoscopy is generally contraindicated with bowel disorders (such as obstruction), cardiorespiratory disease, morbid obesity, increased intracranial pressure, and hypovolemia. During the procedure, insufflation of $CO_2$ to a pressure of 12 to 15 mm Hg (no more than 19 mm Hg) is performed to distend the abdomen (pneumoperitoneum), which causes an increase in $Paco_2$ as $CO_2$ is absorbed, usually plateauing within 10 to 30 minutes. End-tidal $CO_2$ is used to monitor $PaCO_2$, but if comorbidities exist, direct arterial measurement is more accurate. Intrathoracic pressure and systemic vascular resistance may cause an increase in MAP. Preload may decrease with compression of the vena cava. Common issues include increased SVR and left ventricular cardiac stress, decrease in cardiac output, increase in intrathoracic pressure, decrease in vital capacity and decrease in lung compliance. Postoperative nausea and vomiting are common.

## Bariatric surgery

Bariatric surgery is used to promote weight loss in the morbidly obese (100 pounds above normal weight or BMI of 35 to 40). Surgery is performed to restrict intake or prevent absorption of calories. Procedures are open surgical or laparoscopic (most common) with the patient under general anesthesia; they include the following:

- **Banding** places a band around the upper portion of the stomach, creating a small pouch with a small distal opening to slow emptying.
- **Sleeve gastrectomy** removes about two-thirds of the stomach, and a distal part of the small intestine is attached directly to the remaining stomach, bypassing part of the small intestine to reduce absorption.
- **Roux-en-Y** uses staples and a vertical band to decrease the size of the stomach, creating a small pouch. Then a section of the small intestine is attached to the pouch, bypassing the first and second segments of the intestine to reduce absorption.
- **Gastric ballooning** places a balloon in the stomach and fills it with liquid to decrease stomach capacity; this procedure, is used primarily in Europe.

## Breast biopsy

**Breast biopsy** involves removal of tissue to determine whether it is malignant. Biopsy is usually performed for palpable masses, lesions seen on mammography or ultrasound, areas of microcalcifications, changes in the shape of the breast, nipple distortion or discharge, or a recurrent mass at the site of a previous surgical procedure or lesion. Usually, the patient is placed in the supine position and receives local anesthetic, with or without sedation. If the lesion is large and more extensive excision is required (as with lumpectomy), then general anesthesia may be administered. Biopsy may be guided by ultrasonography or mammography. There are several types of biopsies:

- **Fine-needle aspiration** (FNA) uses a needle and syringe to aspirate a small amount of fluid or cells. This technique often yields false-negative results.
- **Excisional biopsy** (lumpectomy) for palpable lesions removes the lesion and surrounding tissue; a frozen section is often examined during surgery.
- **Incisional biopsy** is performed to sample tissue, as when estrogen and progesterone receptors must be examined for recurrent disease.
- **Core needle** (CN) (Tru-Cut) aspiration uses a special large-bore needle and removes one specimen of breast tissue with each needle insertion. It is usually used for large lesions close to the surface and is performed when the lesion is suspected to be carcinoma. The tissue sample is also tested for hormone receptor status.

- *Wire needle localization* uses a long, thin guidewire (placed with guidance by ultrasonography or mammography) inserted through a needle to the area of the lesion before an excisional biopsy is performed so that the surgeon can easily locate the lesion.
- *Vacuum-assisted device* (VAD) may be used to suction a number of tissue samples during one needle insertion.

## Mastectomy

*Mastectomy is surgical removal of* all or part of the breast for treatment (or prophylaxis) of breast cancer. The surgical approach depends on the stage of the cancer:

- 0: Ductal carcinoma in situ (lumpectomy or total mastectomy).
- 1: Lesion 0 to 2 cm in diameter (lumpectomy with axillary lymph node dissection or modified radical mastectomy).
- 2: Lesion 2 to 5 cm lesion in diameter (as for level 1).
- 3: Lesion larger than 5 cm in diameter (modified radical mastectomy)
- 4: Metastasis (possible lumpectomy or modified radical mastectomy)

For surgery the patient is placed in the supine position, and general anesthesia is usually administered, although thoracic epidural anesthesia (TEA) may be used with or without sedation and can be continued by infusion postoperatively to relieve pain. Using TEA rather than volatile anesthetics or opioids reduces the incidence of postoperative nausea and vomiting. TEA may also be used as an adjunct to general anesthesia, providing greater hemodynamic stability by blocking sympathetic nerve fibers.

## Plastic or reconstructive breast surgery

Fewer women undergo mastectomy today because lumpectomy and breast conservation methods have become more widely accepted, but some women who must have or choose mastectomy may also choose to have **breast reconstructive surgery**. Anesthesia and surgery are similar to those used for mastectomy, depending on the type and extent of reconstruction, although different positions may be necessary if flaps are used. Reconstruction may be performed immediately or may be delayed because of radiation or personal choice. Implants are filled with saline (most popular) or silicone gel. Procedures include the following:

- *One-stage:* Immediate insertion of a breast implant during mastectomy if tissue is adequate.
- *Two-stage:* A tissue expander (balloon) with a valve opening to the surface placed beneath the skin. Saline is injected periodically into the expander until the skin has stretched sufficiently. At that point, the expander is removed and an implant is inserted, although some types of expanders can be used as the permanent implant.
- *Tissue flap:* Tissue (skin, muscle, fat, vessels) taken from other areas to make a pedicle or free flap that is shaped into the breast or a pocket for an implant:
- Abdomen (transverse rectus abdominis muscle, TRAM): Uses a pedicle or free flap from the abdomen.
- Abdomen (deep inferior epigastric artery perforator, DIEP): Uses a "tummy tuck" and is a modification of TRAM because only the skin and fat (but no muscle) are used to create an implant pocket.
- Back (latissimus dorsi): A flap from the upper back is tunneled beneath the skin to the chest wall to create a pocket that will hold an implant.

- *Buttocks (gluteal free flap):* Buttocks tissue may be used if the stomach tissue is not adequate.
- ***Nipple/areola reconstruction:*** A final stage (after 3 to 4 months) uses a tissue graft, such as from the other nipple, the ear, the eyelid, or the inner thigh and may involve tattooing to create color for the areola.

### Traumatic amputations and reattachments

**Traumatic amputations** may be partial or complete. The amputated limb should be treated initially as though it could be reattached or revascularized. Single digits, except the thumb, are not usually reattached. Initial treatment includes stabilizing the patient's condition and stopping bleeding by applying a blood pressure cuff proximal to the injury at a pressure 30 mm Hg higher than the systolic pressure for less than 30 minutes. Instruments, such as clamps and hemostats, should be avoided. The stump should be irrigated with normal saline (NS) (not antiseptics) if contaminated. The amputated part should be cooled to 4°C so that the time of viability can be extended and the potential for damage due to ischemia can be reduced. (Single digits and lower limbs are not usually reattached, but the limbs should be treated as though they will be reattached until this determination has been made, especially for children.) The part should be reattached within 6 hours if possible, but reattachment may be delayed for as long as 24 hours if the amputated part is properly cooled. Initial care of an amputated part includes removing jewelry, irrigating the part with NS, and wrapping the part in an NS-moistened dressing (but NOT immersing the part).

### Bone cement implantation syndrome (BCIS)

**Bone cement implantation syndrome** (BCIS) is caused by methyl methacrylate, the cement used to provide fixation of prostheses for joint arthroplasty, particularly hip replacement. The powdered polymerized substance is mixed with a liquid monomer form to create a polymerized form that crosslinks in an exothermic reaction that hardens and expands the cement. This heat, however, causes an expansion of intramedullary gases and increased pressure (>500 mg Hg), which can force embolization of fat, bone marrow, cement, or gas into femoral venous channels. Therefore, nitrous oxide should be discontinued before cement is used. The heat generated may also cause reflex bradycardia, leading to cardiac arrest. Residual liquid monomer can cause vasodilation and decreased vascular resistance. Patients may experience hypotension and hypoxia with dysrhythmias, impaired cardiac output, and pulmonary hypertension. Oxygen administration should be increased before cement is used, adequate fluid volume must be maintained, and central venous pressure (CVP) must be monitored carefully. Cementless prostheses eliminate this complication but require active healthy bones and are contraindicated in the elderly or those with osteoporosis.

### Rotator cuff repair

The **rotator cuff** comprises the muscles and ligaments of the shoulder joint. The bones in the joint include the scapula and the humerus. Muscles (subscapularis, supraspinatus, infraspinatus, and spines minor) and tendons anchor to the head of the humerus so that the arm can move in all directions, and ligaments connect the bones. Part of the rotator cuff is under the scapula. The bursa is between the rotator cuff and the shoulder joint, providing protection. Tears may occur in the ligaments and muscles, and tendonitis or bursitis is also possible. The most common injury to the rotator cuff is a tear in the supraspinatus tendon, so that the tendon is separated from its attachment. Because of lack of adequate blood supply, healing of tears often requires surgical repair. Repair is often done arthroscopically, although open surgery may sometimes be indicated;

- 30 -

the patient is placed in the sitting or lateral decubitus position. Surgery may be performed with the patient under general anesthesia or regional block, such as interscalene.

## Traumatic amputations and reattachment

The amputated part is cooled by placing the wrapped part in a sealed plastic bag and immersing the bag in ice water (1:1 ice-to-water ratio). If the amputation is partial, the treatment is similar, but the NS-wrapped part is splinted, and ice packs or commercial cold packs are applied over the area that is devascularized. Surgical repair, usually performed with the patient under general anesthesia, may require 4 hours or even longer and may involve a number of different surgical teams, depending on the type of amputation and the extent of injury. Regional block with sedation may be used in some cases, such as axillary block for reattachment of fingers. Reattachment is a complicated microsurgical procedure in which bones must be aligned and fixated and vessels, muscles, tendons, ligaments, soft tissue, nerves, and skin must be attached. Heparinization is used to prevent clotting.

## Pneumatic tourniquets

**Pneumatic tourniquets** are frequently used on the upper or lower extremities to decrease blood flow, thereby facilitating surgery. The tourniquet (Esmarch bandage) is typically inflated to 100 mm Hg above the normal systolic BP, but a number of complications are possible, especially when inflation is maintained for more than 2 hours:

- Damage to underlying tissues is possible, including permanent nerve injury. Deep vein thrombosis may occur.
- Posttourniquet syndrome occurs distal to the inflated tourniquet with ischemic changes resulting in lactic acidosis and extracellular potassium, causing changes to capillary permeability. When the cuff is deflated, fluids may move into extracellular spaces, causing edema and compartment syndrome.
- Inflation may cause increased systemic vascular resistance and congestive heart failure. Temperature elevations may occur in children.
- Deflation may cause release of vasoactive metabolic by-products that cause decreased vascular resistance.
- Pain is so severe that regional block may not be adequate for controlling pain. Even under general anesthesia, sympathetic activation may cause hypertension, tachycardia, and diaphoresis.

## Fat embolism

**Fat embolism** can occur when fat enters the venous circulatory system, typically lodging in the pulmonary microvasculature, causing increased pulmonary vascular resistance. Patients most at risk are the young with multiple injuries, the elderly, and those with preexisting disease (pulmonary hypertension, right ventricular disorder, or metastatic cancer). Preventive methods include stabilizing fractures of the long bones or the pelvis within 24 hours of injury. During surgery, with the patient under general anesthesia, fat embolism is indicated by abrupt bradycardia, hypertension, jugular venous distention, hypoxemia, decreased end-tidal $CO_2$ concentration, chest and upper extremity petechiae, fat globules in the retina, and various cardiac irregularities, such as dysrhythmias. Pulmonary artery pressure increases and cardiac output decreases. Right ventricular dysfunction may be evident. Immediate treatment includes 100% oxygen with mechanical ventilation by endotracheal tube (ETT) with adequate IV fluids.

Epinephrine or related drugs may be used for hemodynamic support. In many cases, symptoms are delayed for 1 to 3 days.

### Deep vein thrombosis or thromboembolism

Orthopedic procedures of the pelvis and lower extremities are associated with increased risk of **deep vein thrombosis** (DVT) or **thromboembolism**, especially with older patients, procedures that last longer than 30 minutes, immobilization for more than 4 days, hypothermia, intraoperative hypotension, dehydration, improper positioning that impairs circulation, and use of a pneumatic tourniquet. Stasis, vessel injury, and hypercoagulability (Virchow's triad) promote thromboembolism; therefore, preventive measures include proper positioning, maintaining body heat, providing adequate IV fluids, using intermittent pneumatic compression boots or compression stockings, and medications for reducing coagulopathy (such as heparin). Administration of anticoagulants may be delayed until a few hours postoperatively unless the patient is at risk because of the danger of increased bleeding. Using neuraxial anesthesia alone or in combination with general anesthesia decreases the risk of DVT because of sympathetic activation that increases venous blood flow to the lower extremities. Additionally, local anesthetics increase antiinflammatory effects and reduce platelet reactivity.

### Carpal tunnel release

**Carpal tunnel release** is a common surgical procedure of the upper extremity. Carpal tunnel syndrome is a type of entrapment neuropathy in which the median nerve is compressed by thickening of the flexor tendon sheath, skeletal encroachment, or mass in the soft tissue. Carpal tunnel syndrome is often associated with repetitive hand activities, arthritis, hypothyroidism, diabetes, and pregnancy. Anesthesia is often intravenous regional anesthesia or Bier block. General anesthesia with laryngeal mask airway (LMA) and short-acting anesthetics (propofol and desflurane) may be used. If the operation is prolonged (>1 hr), a brachial plexus block may be chosen, or a field block if a pneumatic cuff is used to reduce bleeding during the operation. The patient is usually supine with the affected arm extended to the side for easy surgical access. A 2- to 3-inch incision is made at the wrist to allow access to the carpal ligament, which is then cut.

### Total hip replacement

**Total hip replacement** is most often indicated for hip fractures associated with osteoarthritis (from repetitive joint trauma), rheumatoid arthritis (from immune-mediated destruction of joints), or osteonecrosis. Rheumatoid arthritis poses particular problems for the anesthetist because multiple joints with severe deformities are usually involved, resulting in difficulty in accessing veins, positioning the patient, and performing intubation. Treatments such as NSAIDs may predispose patients to bleeding. During surgery for total hip replacement, the patient is usually placed in the lateral decubitus position and receives general anesthesia, although neuraxial anesthesia may be used alone or in combination to reduce complications, such as DVT. An incision is made along the lateral thigh so that the femoral head can be removed and the acetabulum reamed in preparation for insertion of the prosthesis. Invasive arterial monitoring is important, especially because of the possibility of bone cement implantation syndrome (BCIS) if the prosthesis is cemented into place.

A number of different procedures may be used for replacement:

- *Posterolateral:* This is the classic approach with a long incision along the hip and lateral thigh.
- *Revision:* This procedure revises a previous procedure, sometimes replacing the entire prosthesis, and may involve substantial loss of blood. In some cases, controlled hypotension is used to reduce bleeding.
- *Minimally invasive procedures* (computer-assisted): These are increasingly used and can allow very accurate placement of prostheses through either one (anterior or posterolateral) or two (anterior and posterior) small incisions. Anesthesia for these procedures is usually epidural (lidocaine 2% and ropivacaine 1%) with propofol infusion and a laryngeal mask airway, with oral opioids for postoperative pain control. Patients can usually leave the hospital within 24 hours.

## Hip fractures

**Hip fractures** most frequently occur in the elderly unless they are associated with serious trauma (as in motor vehicle accidents). Patients may have many comorbid conditions and may present with dehydration and blood loss. Mortality rates are high: 10% during initial treatment and 25% over the next year. Extracapsular fractures (intertrochanteric, subtrochanteric, or base of femoral neck) are associated with more loss of blood than intracapsular fractures (subcapital, transcervical), with which pressure reduces bleeding. Anesthesia may be general or regional (spinal or epidural) or a combination, depending on many variables, such as the patient's cognition and general condition as well as the anticipated length and extent of the surgical procedure. Various types of repair may be performed, including cannulated screw fixation, internal fixation, total hip replacement, extramedullary implant (sliding screw and plate), intramedullary implant (Gamma nail), or hip compression screw and side plate.

## Total knee replacement

Patients who require **total knee replacement** often have profiles to those of patients undergoing total hip replacement, although the surgical procedure is shorter. The knee joint is a hinge joint connecting the femur to the tibia and covered by the patella. A knee prosthesis has three parts: a covering for the end of the femur, a covering for the head of the tibia, and a lining for the patella. A partial knee replacement repairs only one side. Surgery is performed with the patient in the supine position and may require general anesthesia or regional anesthesia with intravenous sedation. Because bone cement implantation syndrome (BCIS) can occur, invasive monitoring of the pulmonary artery and pulmonary artery occlusion pressure (PaOP) is necessary. Additionally, a pneumatic tourniquet is normally used during the procedure to decrease blood loss, posing additional problems, such as hypotension and emboli. Epidural analgesia or insertion of an indwelling femoral sheath catheter may be used to decrease postoperative pain.

## Hemipelvectomy

**Hemipelvectomy** is a radical surgical removal of one leg, the hip joint, and half of the pelvis because of sarcoma (connective tissue cancer). Gluteal muscles that remain are brought around anteriorly and attached to the oblique abdominal muscles to provide some cushioning and support for the operative side, but support for a prosthesis is inadequate and can make fitting difficult; additionally, because sitting upright requires supportive devices, patients need much preoperative support and education. A modified procedure, internal hemipelvectomy, is limb sparing but removes affected areas of the joint and pelvis, sometimes resulting in a flail hip and a 7- to 10-cm difference in leg length. Surgery is often conducted with a combination of general and epidural anesthesia. The duration of surgery varies widely, ranging from 1.5 to 10 hours. Tissue trauma and blood loss are often significant, requiring multiple transfusions and intravenous fluids; therefore, invasive monitoring is critical.

### Vein ligation and stripping

Chronic venous insufficiency results in edema of the lower extremities, causing discomfort and ulcerations. **Ligation and stripping** removes a vein or a section of a vein that is damaged or has damaged valves. An incision below the vein allows an endoscope to be threaded into the vein to grasp and remove (strip) it. The vein is tied (ligated). Sometimes only ligation of a faulty valve is performed, and the vein is left in place. Ligation and stripping is usually performed with the patient under general anesthesia. A number of alternative techniques are performed with the patient under local anesthesia, often in the doctor's office. A newer technique is done with the patient under light anesthesia: transilluminated powered phlebectomy (TIPP). In a darkened operating room, a canula illuminator with a fiberoptic light is fed under the varicose vein through a small incision. Tumescent fluid is infused to loosen attachments and provide local anesthesia. A vein remover, which uses a tiny blade to cut and suction the vein, is inserted through a second incision, guided by the light.

### Transurethral resection of the prostate (TURP)

Benign prostatic hypertrophy or prostatic carcinoma is frequently treated with **transurethral resection of the prostate** (TURP), especially if the volume of the prostate gland reaches only 40 to 50 mL. TURP is performed with the patient in the lithotomy position with legs and feet supported and under general or regional neuraxial anesthesia (spinal or epidural to T10 sensory level) or both. Neuraxial anesthesia provides easier monitoring for complications. A resectoscope is inserted through the urethra, and prostatic tissue is excised with loop and constant irrigation. Complications include TURP syndrome, in which large amounts of fluid ($\geq 2$ L) are absorbed into the venous sinuses and into the systemic circulation, causing hypotension, confusion, cyanosis, pulmonary edema, dyspnea, hyponatremia, excessive blood loss, and seizures because of circulatory overload. Irrigating solutions that contain glycine may cause hyperglycinemia, resulting in CNS toxicity. Other complications include hypothermia, bladder perforation, DIC, and septicemia. Invasive monitoring and evaluation of mental status (in awake patients) are crucial.

### Cystoscopy

**Cystoscopy** may be performed to diagnose the cause of hematuria, recurrent infections, kidney stones, and urinary obstruction. It is also used to facilitate surgical procedures, such as resection of bladder tumors or kidney stones and insertion of ureteral stents, as well as to determine the size of the prostate. Cystoscopy is done with the patient in the lithotomy position, sometimes combined with the Trendelenburg position. Anesthesia may be general, often with a laryngeal mask airway, or regional (spinal and epidural with sensory level to T10). Spinal anesthesia is used more frequently than epidural because of faster onset. Complications are rare because the procedure is usually of short duration; however, perforation of the urethra and scarring can occur. Men may experience testicular swelling and pain after the procedure. Some people experience urinary retention after removal of the cystoscope and may require catheterization; therefore, urinary output should be monitored carefully.

### Dilatation and curettage

**Dilatation and curettage** (D&C) is a procedure in which the cervix is dilated by a series of dilating rods (after insertion of a sound to determine uterine length), and the cervical canal and uterine lining are scraped with a curette, removing the outer layer of abnormal tissue. Although D&C can be performed with the patient under local, spinal, or epidural anesthesia, the procedure is of short duration, so a short-acting general anesthetic is usually administered with the patient in the lithotomy position. This procedure is indicated for diagnosis and treatment of abnormal bleeding or after miscarriage or childbirth to remove remaining tissue. A similar procedure, dilatation and evacuation, uses a vacuum device rather than a curette to remove tissue. Because heavy bleeding may occur in rare cases, fluid balance and blood pressure must be monitored carefully. Complications include perforation of the uterus, bowel, or both, and infection can occur in the postoperative period. Postoperative pain is usually mild, but the patient may experience cramping.

### Pelvic exenteration

**Pelvic exenteration** is a radical removal of pelvic organs (uterus, cervix, vagina, bladder, and rectum) as a treatment for advanced or recurrent cervical, vaginal, rectal, or vulvar cancer in women and for aggressive prostate or rectal cancer in men (includes removal of prostate and associated glands and ducts). Most patients have had previous radiation, chemotherapy, or both. Stoma sites must be identified before surgery, because diversions are necessary after removal of the bladder and rectum. Vaginal reconstruction may be performed with skin grafts. Surgery is performed with the patient in the lithotomy position with careful support of legs and feet to prevent neurological compromise. A number of teams may be involved in the procedure, which can take many hours, posing a challenge to the anesthetist. General anesthesia and epidural may be combined. Invasive monitoring is crucial because there may be substantial blood loss, hypotension, and other complications.

### Hysterectomy

**Hysterectomy** is removal of the uterus and cervix because of uterine bleeding, endometriosis, nonmalignant tumors, or prolapse. A vaginal hysterectomy is contraindicated for large fibroid tumors. Malignancy is most often treated by abdominal hysterectomy with removal of ovaries and fallopian tubes as well. Most simple hysterectomies are done through the vagina, many with laparoscopy, which allows inspection of the abdomen for tumors or abnormalities. During the procedure, the patient is in the lithotomy position. Neuraxial block or general anesthesia (most common) may be used. Another procedure, laparoscopic supracervical hysterectomy (LSH), is a laparoscopic procedure that very small abdominal incisions about the navel and abdomen for insertion of the scope and instruments rather than a vaginal approach. This procedure does not remove the cervix and is less invasive, but the patient must continue with regular Pap smears. In this case, the patient is supine and is placed in the Trendelenburg position.

### Hysteroscopy

**Hysteroscopy** utilizes a hysteroscope, a very thin scope with an attached light and camera, that can pass through the cervix with no or minimal dilation and can provide a view of the inside of the uterus. Carbon dioxide is used to insufflate and expand the uterus for better viewing. Hysteroscopy is usually performed with the patient in the lithotomy position and with a local anesthetic to the cervix, although some additional sedation may be used if the patient is anxious. A somewhat larger hysteroscope may also be used during surgery with either general or regional anesthesia. This scope has channels for microsurgical tools so that biopsies or excisions of polyps, fibroids, or

- 35 -

adhesions can be performed. A resectoscope, used for prostatectomy, can also be used with some modifications for the uterus. This instrument has a dissecting loop that uses an electrical current (high-frequency) for excising and coagulating tissue. Hysteroscopy may be performed to determine the cause of bleeding or infertility.

## Hemorrhoidectomy

**Hemorrhoids** are varicosities of the internal or external hemorrhoidal veins of the anus or rectum. Hemorrhoids may cause severe pain, itching, and bleeding. They are usually caused by straining for a bowel movement, chronic constipation, habitual sitting, or pregnancy. Most treatment is conservative, but surgical repair is necessary if bleeding continues, hemorrhoids prolapse, or pain is severe. Hemorrhoids are classed according to severity:

- First-degree: a hemorrhoid that causes bleeding but does not prolapse.
- Second-degree: a hemorrhoid that prolapses with pressure but then retracts on its own.
- Third-degree: a hemorrhoid that prolapses and must be replaced manually.
- Fourth-degree: a hemorrhoid that prolapses and may thrombose; it cannot be replaced manually.

Surgical procedures are usually performed with the patient in the lithotomy position and under local anesthesia and sedation, although general anesthesia may be used in some cases.

There are many different types of **hemorrhoidectomy**:

- *Sclerotherapy* uses a chemical that is injected about the base of the hemorrhoid, resulting in sclerosing and scarring to replace the hemorrhoid.
- *Infrared coagulation* burns the tissue at the base of the hemorrhoid, forming an eschar that sloughs.
- *Ligation* uses a minute rubber band that is applied to the base of the hemorrhoid by a special "gun" so that the hemorrhoid sloughs.
- *Laser hemorrhoidectomy* vaporizes the hemorrhoid with a focused laser beam and seals off vessels and nerves.
- *Surgical hemorrhoidectomy* may be done by excision of the 3 main hemorrhoidal vessels, leaving 3 pear-shaped areas that are left open to heal or are partially sutured. These procedures are extremely painful and may require weeks for healing.
- *Procedure for prolapse and hemorrhoids (PPH)* (stapling) uses a special circular stapling device to remove excess prolapsed tissue and to staple the remaining tissue to its original position. This is also painful, but less so than traditional surgical repair.
- *Harmonic scalpel hemorrhoidectomy* uses a special ultrasound technology that is similar to laser hemorrhoidectomy but uses lower temperatures and lessens postoperative pain.

## Rectal sphincteroplasty

**Rectal sphincteroplasty** is performed to repair the anal sphincter of patients with fecal incontinence because of damage to the rectal tissue, often caused by an old injury during childbirth. Sphincteroplasty involves a curved incision around the anus, loosening the sphincter muscle and then cutting away weak or damaged muscle from the anal sphincter. The remaining muscle is overlapped and reattached in order to strengthen the sphincter. The bowel is cleansed preoperatively, and diet is restricted to prevent passage of stool to protect the incision from infection during the immediate postoperative period. **Gracilis muscle transplant** uses muscle usually removed from the inner thigh and transplanted to circle the rectal sphincter and provide muscle tone to compensate for loss of nerve function. Postoperative care is similar to that for sphincteroplasty. Sphincteroplasty is performed with the patient in the prone jackknife position under general (most common) or regional anesthesia. Additionally, local anesthetic with epinephrine may be injected to improve hemostasis and relax the muscles.

## Anorectal fistulas (*fistula-in-ano*)

**Anorectal fistulas** extend from the anal canal to the perineal skin. Most originate in the anal glands located between the layers of the anal sphincters and draining into the anal canal. If the glands become blocked and an abscess forms, it can begin to tunnel toward the surface of the skin. There may be only one tunnel or tract or several. Abscesses can become recurrent if they heal over at the surface and purulent material collects, causing pressure to build until it breaks through. Anorectal fistulas are common with Crohn's disease, rectal cancer, or after radiation. Treatment includes antibiotics, Seton (suture holding fistula open) or surgical repair, the most effective treatment but contraindicated for patients with Crohn's disease. Surgical procedures are usually done with the patient under general, spinal, or caudal anesthesia and in the prone jackknife position:

- Fistulotomy is incision of the fistula after the tracts have been identified.
- Fistulectomy is excision of the fistula.

Fistulotomy tends to heal faster than fistulectomy, although recurrence rates are comparable.

## Parks classification of anorectal fistulas

**Parks classification system for anorectal fistulas** classifies 4 different types of cryptoglandular (pertaining to the anal glands) fistulas. The surgical approach may vary somewhat according to the type of anorectal fistula:

- *Intersphincteric* fistulas extend from the internal sphincter downward to the perineum, extend up to a high blind tract, or open into the rectum itself (70%).
- *Transsphincteric* fistulas extend from the internal and external sphincters to the ischiorectal fossa to the perineum (25%).
- *Suprasphincteric* fistulas cross the internal sphincter to the external sphincter above the puborectalis muscles and then down to the ischioanal fossa and to the skin (5%).
- *Extrasphincteric* fistulas extend from the perianal skin through the levator ani muscles and through the rectal wall (1%).

An additional classification is sometimes added to the original 4:

- *Horseshoe* fistulas partially circle the anus, opening at both ends in the cutaneous tissue.

## Orchiectomy

Tumors of the testes may be seminomas or nonseminomas, but the treatment for both involves radical inguinal **orchiectomy**, followed by chemotherapy, radiotherapy, or both, depending on the particular type of tumor. Orchiectomy may be unilateral or bilateral, depending upon the extent of tumor. Surgery is performed with the patient under regional anesthesia, general anesthesia, or both (a combination of general and epidural is common) and with the patient in the supine position. The incision is made parallel and slightly superior to the inguinal ligament on the affected side, and the testicle and spermatic cord are brought through the incision and excised after high spermatic cord ligation. A testicular prosthesis may be placed in the scrotum during the operative procedure. Complications include excessive bleeding and damage to the ilioinguinal nerve, resulting in decreased sensation in the groin and the scrotum on that side. Other surgical treatments (such as scrotal orchiectomy and fine-needle aspiration) are called scrotal violations and may result in disfigurement, although results vary.

## Rhizotomy

**Rhizotomy** is a procedure in which sensory nerve roots are destroyed at the point they enter the spinal cord. A lesion is created that destroys neuronal dysfunction and reduces sensory input. Rhizotomy may be performed as an open procedure (with an incision and clipping of the nerve), percutaneously, or chemically. *Percutaneous trigeminal radiofrequency rhizotomy* relieves the pain associated with trigeminal neuralgia. The rhizotomy needle is inserted into the foramen ovale at the skull base, guided by fluoroscopy or real-time computerized tomographic (CT) fluoroscopy, which provides better visualization. During the procedure, the patient remains awake in the sitting position with intravenous sedation so that the patient can indicate trigeminal paresthesia when the needle is properly placed at the Gasserian ganglion (trigeminal nerve root). The needle electrode is heated while sedation is administered. This procedure provides long-term relief of facial pain but may result in some facial numbness and muscle weakness. A newer procedure uses the Gamma Knife to direct beams of cobalt radiation at the nerve root; this procedure is simple to perform, but pain relief may not be achieved for several weeks.

## Cranioplasty

**Cranioplasty** is repair of a defect or abnormality of the skull, usually with an acrylic plastic plate (methyl methacrylate), although autologous grafts (such as rib grafts) have been used. Autologous grafts are ideal but require an additional surgical procedure and often a different surgeon; therefore, the procedure is more complex. Cranioplasty is performed to improve cosmetic appearance or neurological functioning, such as improving cerebral blood flow, or to prevent further injury. For example, cranioplasty is frequently performed to elevate depressed skull fragments after a skull fracture. General endotracheal anesthesia is usually used, and the positioning of the patient depends on the area of the skull in which the defect occurs. During the procedure, a skin flap is made to expose the underlying skull or tissue. The graft (prefabricated or molded to fit) is secured, usually with stainless steel wire. EEG and invasive monitoring are necessary throughout the procedure.

## Tympanoplasty and mastoidectomy

**Tympanoplasty** is surgical reconstruction of the tympanic membrane. A skin graft is taken from tissue beneath skin about the ear and is used to replace the membrane. If an incision is made behind the ear, the surgical procedure lasts for 2 to 3 hours; if the procedure is performed through the ear canal, it lasts for 30 to 60 minutes. **Mastoidectomy** is an incision into the mastoid cells of the mastoid process because of intractable infection. This procedure is performed only occasionally because more-effective antibiotic therapy is now available. The closed procedure involves an incision behind the ear or through the ear and removes only damaged or infected air cells. More radical procedures may involve removal of the tympanic membrane and most middle ear structures; these procedures resulting in hearing loss. For both procedures, tracheal intubation is performed with an oral or a nasal Ring, Adair, and Elwyn (RAE) tube. Nitrous oxide should be discontinued 30 minutes before the tympanic membrane graft is applied so that pressure against the graft can be prevented, and extubation is performed before the patient emerges to prevent straining. Antiemetics may also be given.

**Middle ear endoscopy, myringotomy, and tympanostomy tube insertion**

**Middle ear endoscopy** may be performed to examine the middle ear. A small-diameter endoscope is used. Usually a topical anesthetic is applied to the tympanic membrane for approximately 10 minutes, and then the external canal is irrigated with normal saline (NS). A small opening is made into the tympanic membrane with a laser or a myringotomy knife, and the endoscope is inserted through the opening.

**Myringotomy**, incision of the tympanic membrane, and insertion of **tympanostomy tubes** for drainage, is a very short procedure (10-15 minutes). It is performed primarily on children who have had repeated episodes of upper respiratory infections and otitis media. Induction is usually with nitrous oxide and halothane with a facemask or laryngeal mask airway (LMA). Intravenous access is not usually required because complications are minimal. Premedication is not usually recommended because the sedation persists longer than the procedure lasts.

**Cataracts**

**Cataracts** are a partial or complete opacity of the lens of one or both eyes; they prevent refraction of light onto the retina. Cataracts can be either congenital or acquired; in children they are associated with prenatal infections such as rubella and cytomegalovirus (CMV) infection, hypocalcemia, and drug exposure. Cataracts can be related to trauma, the administration of systemic corticosteroids, genetic defects (albinism, Down syndrome), and prematurity. Other factors include long-term exposure to sun, family history, and conditions such as diabetes. Age-related cataracts may develop over a number of years. Surgery is usually conducted under local or topical anesthesia, typically a retrobulbar block. A small incision is made into the eye, and the cloudy lens is removed with pulses of liquid or an ultrasonic instrument. The lens is usually replaced with a permanent intraocular acrylic implant. Complications are rare, although bleeding, infection, and retinal detachment can occur.

**Cochlear implant**

A **cochlear implant** is an electronic device that provides sound, although not normal hearing, to those with profound deafness. The person with the implant can often learn to understand speech and environmental sounds. A microphone beside the ear picks up sounds that travels to an external speech processor and transmitter, which sends sounds to an implanted receiver. The receiver converts the sound into electrical impulses that are sent to an internal electrode array implanted in the cochlea. The electrodes send the impulses to the auditory nerve; this creates a perception of sound. Some children now receive bilateral cochlear implants. This procedure (lasting for 3 hours) is performed with the patient under general anesthesia. An incision is made behind the ear, and a depression made in the mastoid process to hold the receiver. An opening is drilled from the mastoid process into the inner ear, and the electrode array is inserted into the cochlea. Glycopyrrolate and fentanyl citrate may be given before induction to prevent postoperative nausea and vomiting.

**Retinal detachment**

The retina is the nerve layer at the posterior inside wall of the eye. It translates light into images. The center, the macula, provides clear images, whereas the rest of the retina provides blurry images. A **retinal detachment** occurs when the retina tears and vitreous fluid leaks through the tear, forcing the retina to separate from the back wall and causing ischemia. Small tears without detachment may be sealed with laser surgery. Anesthesia for retinal detachment repair may be general or regional, such as peribulbar bock. If nitrous oxide is used with general anesthesia, it must be discontinued before the injection of gas to repair the detachment. Procedures include the following:

- **Scleral buckle:** Fluid is drained from the detached area, and a flexible band is placed around the eye to counteract the force that is causing the detachment.
- **Pneumatic retinopexy:** A gas bubble is injected into the vitreous fluid to push the retinal tear against the back wall.
- **Vitrectomy:** Vitreous gel is removed from retina and replaced with a gas bubble. This procedure may be combined with scleral buckle.

## Strabismus

**Strabismus** occurs when the muscles of the eyes are not coordinated and one eye deviates from the axis of the other. Repair is most successful if it is performed when the patient is less than 4 months old, so that stereoscopic vision can remain intact. However, surgery may be performed for cosmetic purposes in older children or adults. Strabismus may be congenital or acquired; it may also be associated with other disorders, such as albinism. Surgical repair of the rectus muscle is performed if conservative treatment (patching, exercises) is ineffective. General anesthesia is used for children, but regional anesthesia, such as retrobulbar block, is used for adults. Retrobulbar block and local infiltration may be used for children in addition to general anesthesia so that postoperative pain can be reduced. One complication of eye surgery is oculocardiac reflex, manifested by bradycardia and other cardiac abnormalities; therefore, an anticholinergic agent (glycopyrrolate) is administered prophylactically before a stimulus that provokes the response (traction on muscles or conjunctiva or placement of retrobulbar block). The risk of hyperthermia and postoperative nausea and vomiting exists.

## Orbital fractures

**Orbital fractures** most often occur with blunt force against the globe, causing a rupture through the floor of the orbital bone, or with a direct blow to the orbital rim, resulting in enophthalmos (sunken globe). Surgical repair is performed approximately about 2 weeks after the injury, when the edema associated with extensive fractures (≥33% of orbital floor) has subsided or when enophthalmos of more than 2 mm and diplopia persist for 10 to 14 days after the injury. Surgical repair is performed with the patient in a sitting position. A combination of local and general anesthesia is usually used. Various surgical approaches, such as transcutaneous or transconjunctival, may be used, depending on the degree of injury. An endonasal approach with an endoscope may also be used to repair injury to the orbital floor. Complications include ischemia of the eye and damage to the optic nerve, resulting in blindness.

## Maxillary fractures

**Maxillary fractures** of the face are often associated with substantial other trauma because of the degree of force necessary to fracture the maxilla. Classifications include the following:

- Le Fort I: horizontal (low downward force)
- Le Fort II: pyramidal (low or mid-maxilla force)
- Le Fort II: transverse (force to bridge of nose or upper maxilla)

However, many injuries consist of more than one type of fracture. With cosmetic surgery, Le Fort fractures may be purposefully created to reshape the face. For traumatic fractures, the patient's airway must remain patent and displaced fragments must be positioned manually. Preinjury photographs should be available to the surgeon as a guide for surgical fixation. Surgery is performed with the patient under general anesthesia and neuromuscular blockade. Orotracheal intubation may be needed if there is intranasal damage, and the position of the tube must be carefully monitored because it may become dislodged as a result of blood, secretions, and repositioning of the head during fixation of the fractures.

## Nasal fracture repair

**Nasal fracture** can result from any type of blunt trauma to the face. This fracture may be overlooked because of edema; therefore, careful examination of the nose is important when a patient presents with facial injuries. The septal cartilage and nasal bones are often fractured. Clear nasal discharge after injury to the face may indicate leakage of cerebrospinal fluid from torn meninges resulting from a fracture of the cribriform plate. A drop of clear drainage should be placed on filter paper and examined for a clear area around a central stain of blood. If CSF drainage is suspected, the patient should be placed upright and should undergo a CT scan; a neurological consult should be requested. Nasal surgery, including elective procedures, is usually done with the patient under local anesthesia and intravenous sedation. Using vasoconstrictors (epinephrine) to reduce bleeding may induce cardiac arrhythmias; therefore, careful monitoring is necessary. Moderate controlled hypotension with slight head elevation may also be used.

## Zygomatic fracture

**Zygomatic fracture** involves the arch of bone that forms the lateral border of the eye orbit and the bony cheek prominence, most commonly associated with a traumatic blow to the lateral cheek. Fracture may change the facial shape, resulting in a tilting of the eye and flattening of the cheek, which may be obscured by initial edema. Fracture may affect only of the arch or may be a more extensive tripod fracture of the infraorbital rim, diastasis of the zygomaticofrontal suture, and disruption of the zygomaticotemporal arch junction. Repair of an uncomplicated fracture of the arch can be performed with the patient under local anesthesia with or without sedation, but repair of tripod fracture requires open reduction with fixation and exploration and reconstruction of the orbit as necessary. This more extensive surgical procedure is usually performed with the patient in the supine position and under local anesthesia, endotracheal general anesthesia, or both.

## Managing increased intracranial pressure

Management of anesthesia for intracranial procedures requires a thorough knowledge of the anesthetic issues related to neurophysiology of the central nervous system, and some anesthetic techniques must be modified because of neurological disorders, such as **increased intracranial pressure** (ICP). Increasing intracranial pressure is a frequent complication of neurological disorders and can indicate cerebral edema, hemorrhage, or obstruction of cerebrospinal fluid. The brain contains 3 compartments: the brain tissue (80%), the cerebrospinal fluid (CSF) (8%), and blood (12%). If normal ICP is to be maintained, a change in volume in one compartment must be compensated for by a reciprocal change in volume in another compartment (*Monroe-Kellie hypothesis*). Normal ICP is 0 to 20 mm Hg with a transducer; increases of more than 30 mm Hg can rapidly decrease cerebral blood flow (CBF), causing ischemia, which further increases ICP, until the cycle results in herniation of the brain, death, or both. *Cushing's triad* is a late sign of increased ICP:

- Increased systolic pressure with widened pulse pressure.
- Bradycardia in response to increased pressure.
- Decreased frequency of respirations.

- 41 -

The brain consumes approximately 20% of the body's oxygen. Cerebral blood flow (CBF) is 750 mL/min, and the brain requires approximately 50 mL for each 100 g of tissue per minute. Cerebral ischemia increases if this amount decreases to less than 25 mL for each 100 g of tissue per minute. The cerebral metabolic rate of oxygen consumption ($CMRo_2$) must be maintained at 3 to 3.5 mL per 100 g of tissue per minute. If the $CMRO_2$ or $Paco_2$ (especially if higher than 50 mm Hg) increases, CBF and ICP increase. Additionally, hyperthermia increases $CMRO_2$ and CBF, and hypothermia decreases both (by 7% for each decrease of 1°C). Anesthetic management includes the following:

- Avoiding premedication that might cause respiratory depression and hypercapnia, which will further increase ICP. Diazepam or midazolam may be used if ICP is within normal range.
- Monitoring direct intraarterial pressure, arterial blood gases, and cerebral blood pressure (zero arterial pressure transducer at head rather than right atrium).
- Using IV agents (barbiturates, propofol, etomidate) that reduce cerebral blood flow and ICP.
- Using intravenous lidocaine, esmolol, labetalol, or a combination of these agents during induction to decrease the risk of hypertension during induction.

### Decompression burr holes

**Decompression burr holes**, circular openings usually made by a craniotome drill (with automatic shut off when tissue is reached), are used to allow access to ventricles for decompression, ventriculography, or shunting procedures. They also provide access for draining abscess or evacuating subdural or extradural hematomas, especially with evidence of increasing intracranial pressure. Burr holes are often used as an emergency treatment before other procedures, such as craniotomy. The area for drilling is shaved and the site is determined, often in the temporal area. A local infiltration of anesthetic, usually containing epinephrine to control bleeding, is used before a 3-cm incision is made to cut through tissue and periosteum. One or more burr holes are drilled, and a closed drainage system is attached. In some cases, the patient may receive general anesthesia for the procedure. Complications include bleeding, infection, and neurological compromise depending on underlying pathology.

### Space-occupying lesions

**Space-occupying lesions** (primary tumors, abscesses, and hematomas) differ according to location, growth rate, and effect on ICP; therefore, careful preoperative evaluation must identify these factors. Premedication is avoided with increased ICP, and invasive monitoring must be continual. Slow induction is often accomplished with hyperventilation and thiopental or propofol, but it varies with the patient's presentation. Patients are usually positioned in the supine position for frontal, temporal, parietal, and occipital lesions with the head raised by 15 to 30 degrees. The patient's head may be turned to the side; therefore, the ETT must be secured, connections must be checked, and the jugular vein must be monitored to ensure that venous flow is not impeded. Because hyperglycemia may increase ischemia, glucose-containing IV fluids are avoided in favor of normal saline (NS) or colloid solutions. Crystalloids in large volumes may increase cerebral edema. Hyperventilation is usually maintained to maintain $Paco_2$ at 30 to 35 mm Hg. Positive end-expiratory pressure (PEEP) should be avoided unless the patient is hypoxic because it may increase ICP. Maintenance usually includes nitrous oxide, opioid, and neuromuscular blocking agents, and emergence must be slow.

### Arteriovenous malformation

**Arteriovenous malformation** (AVM) is a congenital abnormality consisting of a tangle of dilated arteries and veins without a capillary bed. AVMs can occur anywhere in the brain. Usually the AVM

- 42 -

is "fed" by one or more cerebral arteries, which enlarge over time, shunting more blood through the AVM. The veins also enlarge in response to increased arterial blood flow because of the lack of a capillary bridge between the two. Because vein walls are thinner and lack the muscle layer of an artery, the veins tend to rupture as the AVM becomes larger, and a subarachnoid hemorrhage results. Chronic ischemia that may be related to the AVM can result in cerebral atrophy. Treatment may include the following:

- **Radiotherapy** (focused beam) to destroy small AVMs. This is especially useful for AVMs in areas of the brain that are hard to access.
- **Embolization** (percutaneous procedure under fluoroscopic guidance using beads, balloons, or coils to repair the AVM) may be used as an alternative to surgical clipping.

### Space-occupying lesions of the posterior fossa

**Space-occupying lesions of the posterior fossa** pose challenges. The patient may be in the modified lateral, prone, or sitting position, with the head elevated. If the patient is in a sitting semirecumbent position, the head is fixed in a holder with the neck flexed, although excessive flexion must be avoided. Complications include the following:

- Hydrocephalus caused by from obstruction of CSF at the 4th ventricle (resulting in increased ICP), requiring ventriculostomy before induction.
- Pneumocephalus (especially when the patient is in a sitting position) as air replaces lost CSF.
- Brain stem injury resulting from surgical trauma, especially affecting the cardiopulmonary system.
- Venous air embolism (especially when the patient is in a sitting position). Small venous air emboli are absorbed through the respiratory system, but large emboli can overwhelm the system, decreasing cardiac output. Because this effect is magnified by nitrous oxide, this agent is often avoided when patients are in a sitting position; alternatively, the concentration is decreased to 50%. Right atrial catheterization facilitates aspiration of entrained air and is frequently used for patients in a sitting position. TEE and precordial Doppler sonography monitor patients for venous air embolism.

### Cerebral aneurysm

Surgical **clipping** of a ruptured **cerebral aneurysm** within 48 hours of rupture is necessary to reduce the risk of rebleeding, which is 4% during the first 24 hours and 1% to 2% per day for the next month. Clipping may be performed prophylactically to prevent rupture. Clipping secures the aneurysm without impairing circulation. When bleeding is controlled, a small spring-like clip or multiple clips are placed about the neck of the aneurysm. The bulging part of the aneurysm is aspirated to ensure that it does not refill, and angiography may be performed to ensure patency of the artery that feeds the aneurysm. During surgery, a clot may break away from the aneurysm, resulting in extensive hemorrhage. Neurological damage may occur because of surgical manipulation. Controlled hypotension is sometimes used to decrease arterial pressure and lessen the danger of rebleeding; however, blood must be available for transfusion. Anesthetic goals are to prevent increased pressure and rupture or rebleeding. Mannitol may be used after the dura has been opened to reduce trauma.

## Arteriovenous malformation

*Surgical excision of AVM* is the definitive treatment for AVMs because both embolization and radiotherapy pose a risk of recurrence of the abnormal vessels. Sometimes, 2 or 3 surgical procedures may be required to correct large AVMs. Usually, AVMs are surrounded by nonfunctioning brain tissue; therefore, it is possible to remove them without damaging brain tissue. However, reperfusion bleeding may occur as blood is diverted to surrounding arteries that had dilated because of chronic ischemia. The sudden increase in blood flow and pressure may cause leakage of blood from the vessels. Blood loss during surgery may be extensive; therefore, constant monitoring of arterial pressure and the use of multiple IV cannulas are important. Embolization may be performed before surgery to reduce bleeding. Hyperventilation and mannitol are often used, and β-blockers may be used to prevent hypertension and cerebral edema. Postoperatively, blood pressure is kept low to prevent reperfusion bleeding.

## Transorbital approach

The **transorbital approach** for intracranial surgery is used for brain, sinus, and orbit procedures, obviating the need to remove a large section of frontal bone to access the brain. This procedure is used for meningioma, hemangioma, pituitary adenoma, schwannoma, and other types of lesions. It provides easy access to optic and skull base lesions. A number of procedures are possible, but the supraorbital requires a small incision over the eyebrow, with removal of a small portion of the frontal bone and the orbit. Magnetic resonance imaging (MRI) guidance and microsurgical techniques are used to locate and excise or repair the lesion. Incisions may also be made below the brow or eye or at the medial or lateral aspects, depending on the location and extent of the lesion. The patient receives general anesthesia and is usually supine, with the head turned to the nonoperative side to allow easy access to the surgical site; therefore, the head must be carefully positioned so that vascular occlusion can be prevented.

## Transsphenoidal hypophysectomy

The sella turcica is a depressed area that holds the pituitary gland (which extends down from the brain on a stalk) in the sphenoid bone at the base of the skull. A pituitary tumor less than 10 mm diameter is removed by **transsphenoidal hypophysectomy**. The patient is supine, with the head slightly elevated. General anesthesia is achieved with an endotracheal tube. Supplemental infraorbital blocks may provide postoperative pain relief. Vasoconstrictors (such as epinephrine) with local anesthesia are usually administered intranasally to control bleeding. Microscopic surgery is performed with an incision in the gingival mucosa beneath the upper lip and then through the nasal septum and the roof of the sphenoid cavity to access the base of the sella turcica and the pituitary tumor. Endoscopic surgery is performed directly through the nares with removal of mucosa but no incision. After microscopic surgery, stents are placed in the nasal septum, and the nose is packed. With both procedures, nasal discharge must be observed for CSF leakage, and the patient must be cautioned not to blow the nose.

## Stereotactic procedures (CyberKnife)

**CyberKnife** is a frameless **stereotactic radiosurgery** device that provides results similar to those achieved with the Gamma Knife but uses a wire-mesh face mask or body immobilizer rather than a frame for precise targeting. It is used for both benign and malignant tumors, especially those of the spine and spinal cord, intracranial lesions, pancreatic and adrenal tumors, AVMs, and hepatocellular cancer. Physicians can more easily divide a large radiosurgical dose into more than one stage or fraction, called staged radiosurgery, because there is no need to attach a frame before each treatment. The CyberKnife system uses a miniature linear accelerator mounted on a flexible, robotic arm and a 6D system, which corrects for 6 motions (3 translational motions and 3 rotational), using the skeleton as a frame of reference. Intracranial surgery may require implantation of radiopaque markers. An image-guidance system tracks the target location during treatment to allow for accuracy to 0.5 mm. Some patients may experience transient dizziness, lightheadedness, or mild headaches after treatment; in such cases, a course of corticosteroids is required.

### Stereotactic procedures (Gamma Knife)

**Stereotactic radiosurgery** uses focused radiation to treat brain tumors. The **Gamma Knife,** used for tumors less than 4 cm in diameter, is one type of stereotactic radiosurgery. Before the procedure, the patient is fitted with a stereotactic frame, which, after the administration of a local anesthetic, is screwed to the skull to immobilize the head. Using computed tomography (CT) and MRI, a 3D image of the brain is created, which allows the physician to locate the tumor, a process that may take as long as 5 hours. The patient is then placed in a metal helmet-like device with several ports through which 201 beams of cobalt 60 are directed at the lesion's center. At the point at which the 201 beams cross, enough radiation is delivered to affect the tissue, but the surrounding healthy tissue is not damaged. The treatment continues for 3 to 10 minutes. Some tumors require more than one treatment. Children may require general anesthesia, and some adults may need sedation. There is some risk of radiation necrosis with all types of radiosurgery.

### Bronchoscopy

**Bronchoscopy** uses a thin flexible fiberoptic bronchoscope to inspect the larynx, trachea, and bronchi for diagnostic purposes. It is also used to collect specimens, obtain biopsies, remove foreign bodies or secretions, treat atelectasis, and excise lesions. The patient is in the supine position during the procedure. The Mallampati classification may be used to determine the difficulty of the airway. The patient receives local anesthesia to the nares (lidocaine gel) and oropharynx (lidocaine gel, spray, or nebulizer), and usually receives a benzodiazepine (commonly midazolam or lorazepam), an opioid (fentanyl or meperidine), or propofol. Medications are usually given in small incremental doses throughout the procedure and may be combined. Oversedation may cause physiologic depression, but undersedation may result in recall and agitation with sympathetic activation. The tube is advanced through the nares and down the trachea to the bronchi. Airway patency, respiratory rate, and oxygen saturation must be constantly monitored. Complications can include bleeding, arrhythmias, obstruction, laryngospasm, and respiratory failure.

### Esophagogastroduodenoscopy

**Esophagogastroduodenoscopy** is performed with a flexible fiberscope equipped with a lighted fiberoptic lens to allow direct inspection of the mucosa of the esophagus, stomach, and duodenum. The scope is equipped with a still or video camera attached to a monitor for viewing during the procedure. The scope may be used for biopsies and also therapeutically to dilate strictures or treat gastric or esophageal bleeding. This procedure is usually performed with the patient on the left side (with the head supported) to allow drainage of saliva. Conscious sedation (midazolam) is commonly used along with a topical anesthetic spray or gargle to facilitate placing the lubricated tube through the mouth into the esophagus. Atropine may be given to reduce secretions. A bite guard is placed into the mouth to prevent the patient from biting the scope. The airway must be carefully monitored throughout the procedure (which usually lasts approximately 30 minutes); an oximeter must be used to measure oxygen saturation.

### Oropharyngeal reconstruction

**Oropharyngeal reconstruction** may be necessary after radical removal of tumors or after radiotherapy. Patients are evaluated with videofluoroscopy (VFS) for ability to swallow, to identify interventions, and for fiberoptic endoscopic evaluation of swallowing (FEES) to show the effects below the mouth, including evidence of aspiration. These tests can identify tongue movement, laryngeal and epiglottis position during swallowing, and sphincter activity. Reconstruction may involve placement of prosthesis, bone grafts, and flaps. Axial or free flaps are used for reconstruction of large defects. Axial flaps are rotated to the site from adjacent tissue and have a vascular system along the axis of the tissue. Axial flaps can include myocutaneous flaps (usually pectoralis or trapezius) with skin and subcutaneous fat and muscle. Free flaps (such as radial forearm) are taken from a nonadjacent body area and attached microvascularly. In some cases, vascular reconstruction must be completed and autologous vein or artery grafts must be used. The patient is supine and receives general anesthesia, sometimes combined with regional anesthesia.

### Hyoid fracture

The **hyoid** bone is located above the larynx and is not attached to other bones but is held in place by ligaments attached to processes of the temporal bones of the skull. The hyoid bone provides support for the tongue and attaches a number of different muscles that control movement of the larynx, speech, and swallowing. This horseshoe-shaped bone is relatively flexible in children and adolescents but can break in adults. A fracture in the hyoid bone may be found with adult victims of strangulation or rarely as the result of other direct trauma. In most cases, nonstrangulation fractures are accompanied by multiple other facial or oropharyngeal fractures, such as pharyngeal or laryngeal, and hyoid fracture may be overlooked. Management of hyoid fractures alone is usually conservative, but in some cases, such as with perforation of the pharynx or multiple fractures, surgical repair with general anesthesia may be indicated.

### Dental surgery

Although most **dental surgery,** such as removal of wisdom teeth, is performed with the patient under local anesthetic, children, mentally handicapped patients, or adults who are fearful of dental procedures may require general anesthesia. Induction is commonly performed with ketamine IM, after which an intravenous line is placed and IV anesthetic agents are administered, including thiopental, etomidate, or propofol. Alternately, inhalation anesthesia (sevoflurane) may be used. If the procedure may involve considerable blood loss, then atropine may be administered. Nasal intubation with a cuffed endotracheal tube is recommended for long procedures. Different drugs are used for maintenance, depending on the duration of surgery. These may be a combination of both inhaled and IV drugs. Opioids, such as remifentanil and alfentanil, may be used because they are short-acting. Airway patency must be monitored continually, especially during emergence if there is oropharyngeal packing or bleeding.

### Tonsillectomy and adenoidectomy

**Tonsillectomy and adenoidectomy** may be performed to treat recurrent infections but are most often performed for hyperplasia and obstructive sleep apnea (OSA). Surgery should be delayed if infection is present. Preoperative sedation may be avoided for children with OSA or severe hyperplasia, and, in those cases, inhalational induction and establishment of positive-pressure ventilation should be performed before neuromuscular blocking agents are administered. A reinforced Ring, Adair, and Elwyn (RAE) right-angled endotracheal tube may be used with extubation after the patient emerges. The patient is supine with the neck hyperextended (supported) and the mouth braced open. Bleeding and aspiration are possible complications; therefore, the patient must be monitored carefully, and intravascular volume must be maintained. The patient should be placed in a non-supine position and carefully observed in the recovery area for evidence of bleeding that may require nasogastric (NG) tube, volume replacement, rapid-sequence induction, and surgical control of bleeding. Adenoidectomy may be done alone by endoscopic nasal surgery with the patient under general anesthesia.

## Orthodontic

**Orthodontic** surgery, ***orthognathy***, corrects misalignment of jaws or teeth that causes dental, swallowing, or cosmetic problems. A prognathic jaw protrudes, and a retrognathic jaw recedes. Preoperative evaluation of the airway is important, because multiple problems may exist that could interfere with intubation or mask ventilation. In some cases, fiberoptic oral intubation or nasal RAE tube may be necessary. The patient receives general anesthesia while in the supine position with the head slightly elevated to reduce bleeding. Local infiltration with epinephrine and controlled hypotension may also be used because this area is vascular, and blood loss may be substantial. At least two intravenous lines must be placed before surgery, and an oropharyngeal pack may be placed to prevent blood and other debris from entering the larynx and trachea. End-tidal $CO_2$ and peak inspiratory pressure should be carefully monitored throughout the procedure. The packing is removed at the end of the procedure, and the pharynx is carefully suctioned. Extubation is performed upon full emergence if there is no bleeding.

## Pharyngoplasty

**Pharyngoplasty** is primarily performed to correct velopharyngeal dysfunction (VPD), in which the velopharyngeal sphincter, situated between the oral and nasal cavities, does not function properly. The VP sphincter controls the flow of air through the chambers, modulating the voice, and prevents backflow and regurgitation into the nasal cavity from the oral cavity. Therefore, it is essential for swallowing. Incompetence of the sphincter may relate to congenital defects, such as cleft palate, but may also relate to myoneural or behavioral disorders. VPD may occur with myasthenia gravis, cerebrovascular accident (CVA), or lesions of motor neurons. Nasoendoscopic and fluoroscopic speech and swallowing evaluations are performed preoperatively. A pharyngeal flap from the posterior wall of the pharynx is attached to the soft palate, leaving small bilateral openings (ports) that open and close with respirations and voicing. Prostheses are also available and can be used successfully, but compliance is often poor. Surgery is performed with the patient under general anesthesia and with careful monitoring of the airway.

## Rigid laryngoscopy

Flexible laryngoscopy is usually performed through the nares with a local anesthetic in the nose and throat while the patient is awake, often in a sitting or reclining position. In this way, the vocal cords can be examined while the patient speaks. However, a **rigid laryngoscope** is commonly used during surgical procedures with the patient under general anesthesia, often in conjunction with topical lidocaine, with the patient in the supine position. The laryngoscope with a blade, handle, and light is also used by the anesthetist for intubation. The physician may use one of approximately a dozen specialized types of rigid laryngoscope, depending on the purpose. The laryngoscope is inserted through the mouth and allows the surgeon to examine the larynx and vocal cords, remove foreign objects or polyps, take a biopsy specimen, or perform laser treatments. The surgeon can look directly through the laryngoscope or can attach a still or video camera, connected to a monitor, for magnified viewing.

### Intraaortic balloon pump

**The intraaortic balloon** (IAB) pump is the most commonly used circulatory assist device. It is used for a number of problems (unstable angina, myocardial infarction, cardiogenic shock, papillary muscle dysfunction, ventricular failure after cardiac surgery, and dysrhythmias) and may be used to facilitate weaning patients from CPB after open-heart surgery if the heart is not able to pump adequately. The IAB consists of a 90-cm stiff catheter with a 25-cm inflatable balloon from the tip and lengthwise down the catheter. The catheter is usually inserted through the femoral artery but may be placed during surgery or through a cutdown. The catheter is threaded into the descending thoracic aorta, and the balloon inflates during diastole to increase circulation to the coronary arteries; it then deflates during systole to decrease afterload. Complications can include dysrhythmias, peripheral ischemia from femoral artery occlusion, and balloon perforation or migration. Tachycardia and dysrhythmias may interfere with timing the pump.

### Cardiopulmonary bypass

Open-heart surgical procedures require **cardiopulmonary bypass** (CPB) or extracorporeal circulation. Premedication includes benzodiazepines (midazolam, diazepam, or lorazepam) alone or with an opioid, such as morphine. The patient should be preoxygenated before induction with IV anesthetics, and intubation should be performed quickly to avoid stimulation that may affect hemodynamics. Nitrous oxide is avoided so that intravascular air bubbles can be prevented. Monitoring includes the following:

- Urinary output, blood pressure, arterial blood gas, pH, electrolytes, clotting times, ECG (especially leads II and $V_5$ to check for dysrhythmias and ischemic changes), transesophageal echocardiography (TEE), and transcranial Doppler.
- A pulmonary artery catheter should be in place for cardiac monitoring to allow evaluation of right and left ventricular volumes and functions and valvular functions.
- Both core temperature and skin temperature should be monitored. Hypothermia will be used to lower $O_2$ demand.

Anesthesia should be deep before sternotomy so that stimulation can be avoided, and the patient should be hand-ventilated during this part of the procedure so that trauma to the lungs can be prevented. The patient is heparinized approximately 3 minutes before CPB and insertion of cannulas so that clotting can be prevented.

A return cannula is usually placed in the ascending aorta but may be placed in the femoral artery. A cross-clamp is placed across the aorta (below the return cannula) to divert blood to the bypass machine. (The lungs are not mechanically ventilated during CPB.) The blood drains from the cannulas into a venous reservoir and then is pumped through a filter that removes air bubbles or clots. After filtering, the blood is oxygenated by a membrane-gas-interface to maintain the $Pao_2$ with $Paco_2$ at 35 to 45 mm Hg. The blood goes through a heat exchanger to heat or cool the blood, depending on the stage of the operation. Temperature is usually maintained at 18°C before arrest and at 28° to 32° during surgery; it is then increased to 37° before removal from the bypass machine. Cooled blood is more viscous, but it is diluted by crystalloid solutions (commonly 5% dextrose in lactated Ringer's). The blood is then pumped back into the circulation, bypassing the heart.

Cardiopulmonary bypass care should be aimed at protecting the renal and hepatic systems during surgery, and preventing nervous system or cardiac injury. Before placing a patient on CPB the patient must have adequate anesthesia, A-line monitoring of blood pressures, core temperature

- 48 -

monitoring, ACT at least 400, satisfactory arterial inflow of oxygenated blood, and adequate venous return to the bypass pump.

Activated coagulation time (ACT) is checked before heparin is administered, after CPB is initiated, 3 minutes after heparin is administered, after each incremental dose, and every 30 to 60 minutes. ACT is usually maintained at more than 400 to 480 seconds. After the heart is accessed through a midsternal incision and sternotomy, a single cannula is placed into the right atrium or the femoral vein, or dual catheters are placed through the right atrium into the superior and inferior vena cava to provide gravity drainage of venous blood, because the pump system creates a vacuum. (If the aortic valve is incompetent, then the left ventricle must be vented to prevent backflow of blood into the left ventricle.) Note:

- Improper placement of the superior vena cava cannula can result in increased central venous pressure (CVP) and cerebral edema, and improper placement of the inferior vena cava cannula can cause abdominal vascular distention with inadequate venous return to the CPB machine.

**Cardiopulmonary bypass (Anesthetic protocols)**

Cardioplegic potassium-based solution is infused into the aortic root, from which it circulates to the coronary arteries, to ensure cessation of electrical activity so that the heart remains flaccid during CPB. However, this infusion can result in postoperative hyperkalemia, although excess potassium can be filtered by the CPB machine. Anesthetic agents used for CPB may vary, but NMBAs, such as rocuronium or vecuronium, are necessary with other agents. Commonly used **protocols** include the following:

- Total intravenous anesthesia with short-acting agents (such as propofol and remifentanil or morphine) to allow early extubation.
- Mixed intravenous and inhalation anesthesia with propofol, etomidate or thiopental, and midazolam for induction. Volatile agents (isoflurane, desflurane, or sevoflurane) and opioids (remifentanil or propofol) are used for maintenance.
- Combined ketamine and midazolam for induction and maintenance with propofol during induction and a volatile agent added during maintenance. (Often used for frail patients, but may prolong emergence.)

**Cardiopulmonary bypass (Discontinuation)**

To **discontinue CPB**, the patient must be rewarmed, air must be evacuated from the system, the aortic cross-clamp must be opened and removed, and mechanical ventilation must be restarted. Guidelines for discontinuation include the following:

- Core temperature should be 37°C to prevent metabolic acidosis and decreased myocardial contractility.
- Cardiac status must be stable with sinus rhythm (preferable) and evidence of AV block. In some cases, increased potassium levels must be treated with calcium, furosemide, or glucose and insulin. AV pacing may be required. Heart rate should be 80 to 100 bpm. Bradycardia may be treated with pacing or inotropic agents. Cardioversion may be necessary if supraventricular tachycardia occurs. Perfusion should be adequate.
- Laboratory values must be checked and must be within normal limits: hematocrit, 22% to 25%; potassium, <5.5 mEq/L; and pH, >7.20.

- Monitors must be functioning properly.
- Ventilation is resumed with 100% oxygen.

The patient is weaned slowly from CPB. If pump failure occurs as CPB is discontinued, an intraaortic balloon pump may be used before another attempt is made to wean the patient.

### Repair of cardiac valves

A number of different surgical options are available for **repair of cardiac valves**:

- *Valvotomy/Valvuloplasty* is usually performed through cardiac catheterization. A valvotomy/valvuloplasty may involve releasing valve leaflet adhesions that interfere with functioning of the valve. In balloon valvuloplasty, a catheter with an inflatable balloon is positioned in the stenotic valve and inflated and deflated a number of times to dilate the opening.
- *Aortic valve replacement* is an open-heart procedure with cardiopulmonary bypass. Aortic valves are tricuspid (3 leaflets); because repair is usually not possible, defective valves must be replaced with either mechanical (metal, plastic, or pyrolytic carbon) or biological (porcine or bovine xenografts) valves.
- *Aortic homograft* uses part of a donor's aorta with the aortic valve attached to replace the recipient's faulty aortic valve and part of the ascending aorta.
- *Ross procedure* uses the patient's pulmonary artery with the pulmonary valve to replace the aortic valve and part of the aorta and then uses a donor graft to replace the pulmonary artery.

### Anesthesia management of aortic surgery

Most patients presenting for aortic surgery have multiple comorbidities that significantly alter outcomes. Preexisting heart disease is the main risk factor for mortality in the perioperative period for a patient having aortic surgery. Goals of anesthesia in this patient population include:

- Maintain intravascular volume
- Control heart rate and afterload
- Replace blood loss aggressively, monitoring for coagulopathy if large loss
- Control blood glucose to prevent ketoacidosis and improve outcomes
- Avoid hypoperfusion during aortic cross-clamping
- Before unclamping, IV fluid bolus is commonly given

Postoperative renal failure can have a huge impact on patient outcomes. To preserve renal function, focus on maintaining fluid volume, renal perfusion, and cardiac output. The best indicator of postop renal issue is having pre-op renal disease. It is important to maximize renal function before surgery. Especially in patients with pre-op renal disease, nephrotoxic drugs and drugs that decrease blood flow to the kidney should be avoided. Minimizing cross-clamp time is important in decreasing chances of renal dysfunction, among other complications. Maintaining anesthesia and analgesia is very important in this patient population and muscle relaxation is important as well. There are advantages to using epidural analgesia, as it decreases sympathetic nervous system tone, preventing or decreasing high blood pressure and tachycardia, thus decreasing cardiac workload. Epidural must be placed at least one hour prior to heparinizing the patient, due to issues with hematoma formation.

## Coronary artery bypass grafting (CABG)

**Coronary artery bypass grafting (CABG)** is a surgical procedure for treatment of angina that does not respond to medical treatment, unstable angina, blockage of more than 60% in the left main coronary artery, blockage of multiple coronary arteries (including the proximal left anterior descending artery), left ventricular dysfunction, and previous unsuccessful attempts to perform percutaneous coronary intervention (PCI). The surgery is performed through a midsternal incision that exposes the heart, which is chilled and placed on cardiopulmonary bypass with blood going from the right atrium to the machine and back to the body; the aorta is clamped to keep the surgical field free of blood. Bypass grafts are sutured into place to bypass areas of occluded coronary arteries. Grafts may be obtained from various sites:

- Gastroepiploic artery.
- Internal mammary artery (commonly used and superior to saphenous vein but procedure is more time-consuming).
- Radial artery.
- Saphenous vein (commonly used, especially for emergency procedures).

## Minimally-invasive direct coronary artery bypass (MIDCAB)

**Minimally-invasive direct coronary artery bypass (MIDCAB)** applies a bypass graft on the beating heart through a 10-cm incision in the mid-chest rather than midsternally, without using cardiopulmonary bypass. Because the incision must be over the bypass area, this procedure is suitable for bypass of only one or two coronary arteries. A small portion of rib is removed to allow access to the heart, and the internal mammary artery is used for grafting. Special instruments, such as a heart stabilizer, are used to limit movement of the heart during suturing. The procedure usually lasts for 2 to 3 hours, and recovery time is decreased because patients experience less pain. Because anastomosis is difficult when the heart is beating, complications such as ischemia may occur during surgery; therefore, a cardiopulmonary bypass machine must be available. Early studies indicate that MIDCAB may provide longer-lasting relief than angioplasty for single-vessel occlusion.

## Port access coronary artery bypass grafting

**Port access coronary artery bypass grafting** is an alternative form of CABG that uses a number of small incisions (ports) along with cardiopulmonary bypass (CPB) and cardioplegia to perform a video-assisted surgical repair. Usually 3 or more incisions are required, with one in the femoral area to allow access to the femoral artery for a multipurpose catheter that is threaded through to the ascending aorta to return blood from the CPB, block the aorta with a balloon, provide cardioplegic solution, and vent air. Another catheter is threaded through the femoral vein to the right atrium to carry blood to the CPB. An incision is also needed for access to the jugular vein for catheters to the pulmonary artery and the coronary sinus. One to three thoracotomy incisions are made for insertion of video imaging equipment and instruments. Although the midsternal incision is avoided, multiple incisions pose the potential of possible morbidity.

## Percutaneous transluminal coronary angioplasty (PTCA)

**Percutaneous transluminal coronary angioplasty (PTCA)** is an option for poor surgical candidates who have an acute MI or uncontrolled chest pain. This procedure is usually performed only to increase circulation to the myocardium by breaking through an atheroma if there is collateral circulation. The patient receives IV sedation and local anesthesia. A hollow catheter (sheath) is inserted, usually from the femoral vein or artery, and is fed through the vessels to the coronary arteries. When the atheroma is verified by fluoroscopy, a balloon-tipped catheter is fed over the sheath, and the balloon is inflated with a contrast agent to a specified pressure to compress the atheroma. The balloon may be inflated a number of times to ensure that residual stenosis is less than 20%. Laser angioplasty using the excimer laser is also used to vaporize plaque. **Stents** may be inserted during the angioplasty to maintain vessel patency. Stents may be flexible plastic or wire mesh and are typically placed over the catheter, which is inflated to expand the stent against the arterial wall.

### Directional coronary atherectomy (DCA), rotational atherectomy (ROTA), and transluminal extraction

**Directional coronary atherectomy (DCA)** is the removal of an atheroma from an occluded coronary artery. The patient receives IV sedation and local anesthesia. This procedure may be more effective than angioplasty because it shaves an atheroma away instead of compressing it. Sometimes angioplasty is the first step in DCA if the vessel is too narrow for the DCA catheter; it is the last step if the tissue needs smoothing. The DCA catheter is a large balloon catheter that is usually inserted over a sheath through the femoral artery. The catheter includes an open window on one side of the balloon with a rotational cutting piston that shaves the atheroma with the plaque residue pushed inside the device for removal. The procedure may require 4 to 20 cuts, depending on the extent of the plaque. A similar procedure is **rotational atherectomy (ROTA),** which uses a catheter with a diamond-chip drill at the tip; the drill rotates at 130,000 to 180,000 RPM, pulverizing the atheroma into microparticles. A **transluminal extraction** catheter uses a motorized cutting head with a suction device for residue.

### Transmyocardial laser revascularization (TMR)

**Transmyocardial laser revascularization** is performed percutaneously or through a midsternal or thoracotomy incision. The patient receives general anesthesia (or local anesthesia and sedation for percutaneous procedure), but CPB is not needed unless this procedure is combined with coronary bypass surgery:

- Percutaneously, a fiberoptic catheter is positioned inside the ventricle and against the ischemic area. Laser bursts are used to cut 20 to 40 channels into but not through the myocardium. The laser burns create channels and stimulate an inflammatory response, which causes new blood vessels to form (angiogenesis), thereby improving circulation to the myocardium and reducing ischemia and pain.
- Surgically, the catheter tip is positioned on the outside of the left ventricle rather than on the inside while the heart is beating without bypass.

These procedures do not affect mortality rates but do reduce symptoms and increase tolerance to activity, thereby improving the quality of life. Postoperative care for the percutaneous procedure is the same as that for percutaneous transluminal coronary angioplasty (PTCA), whereas care for the surgical procedure is similar to that for coronary artery bypass grafting (CABG).

### Aortic aneurysm

An **aortic aneurysm** occurs when a weakness in the wall of the aorta causes a ballooning dilation of the wall of the aorta. There are a number of types:

- *False*: Caused by a hematoma that may pulsate and erode the vessel wall.
- *True*: Bulging involves 1 to 3 layers of the vessel wall.

- 52 -

- *Fusiform:* Symmetric bulging about the entire circumference of vessel.
- *Saccular:* Ballooning on one side of vessel wall.
- *Dissecting:* Occurs when the wall of the aorta is torn and blood flows between the layers of the wall, dilating and weakening it until it risks rupture (90% mortality rate).

The *DeBakey classification* uses anatomic location as the focal point:

- *Type I* begins in the ascending aorta but may spread to include the aortic arch and the descending aorta (60%). (Proximal or Stanford type A lesion.)
- *Type II* is restricted to the ascending aorta (10% to 15%). (Proximal or Stanford type A).
- *Type III* is restricted to the descending aorta (25% to 30%). (Distal or Stanford type B).

Surgery for the ascending aorta and aortic arch are performed with median sternotomy and cardiopulmonary bypass (CPB) with hypothermia. Anesthetic management is similar to that for other CPB procedures. The patient is in the supine position and receives general intubated anesthesia. There may be numerous complications, including excessive blood loss, extended cross-clamp time, and aortic regurgitation. In some cases, aortic valve replacement must be performed as part of surgical repair. Anesthetic management includes the following:

- Monitoring: multiple invasive with transesophageal echocardiography (TEE), arterial blood pressure (left radial artery), EEG.
- Blood pressure control with nitroprusside to prevent hypotension.
- β-blocker (esmolol) is used with aortic dissection.
- CPB arterial inflow must be placed in the femoral artery with dissection.
- Hypothermia (to 15°C) is necessary for aortic arch surgery so that cerebral damage can be prevented. This is combined with thiopental infusion. Steroids may also be administered.

## Atrial septal defect

An **atrial septal defect (ASD)** is an abnormal opening in the septum between the right and left atria. It is often congenital, but it may not be apparent until childhood or adulthood (in rare cases). Because the left atrium has higher pressure than the right atrium, some of the oxygenated blood returning from the lungs to the left atrium is shunted back to the right atrium, where it is again returned to the lungs, displacing deoxygenated blood. Symptoms depend on the degree of the defect but can include congestive heart failure, heart murmur, and increased risk of dysrhythmias and pulmonary vascular obstructive disease. Surgery may not be necessary for small defects, but larger defects require closure:

- Open-heart surgical repair may be done with general anesthesia and CPB.
- An alternative procedure is minimally invasive cardiac catheterization and placement of a closure device (Amplatzer device, a septal occluder) across the atrial septal defect. This procedure is performed with general anesthesia for children and local anesthesia and sedation for adults.

## Atrioventricular canal defect

**Atrioventricular canal defect** is often associated with Down syndrome (trisomy 21) and involves a number of defects, including openings between the atria and ventricles and abnormalities of the valves. In partial defects consist of an opening between the atria with mitral valve regurgitation. In complete defects, there is a large central hole in the heart and only one common valve between the atria and ventricles. The blood may flow freely about the heart, usually from left to right. Extra

- 53 -

blood flow to the lungs causes enlargement of the heart and typical symptoms of congestive heart failure and lung disease, with increasing dyspnea and cyanosis. Partial defects may go undiagnosed for 20 years. Open-heart surgery with CPB and general anesthesia is performed to patch holes in the septum (often using a graft from the pericardial sac) and to repair or replace valves. The procedure is usually performed by the time the infant reaches 6 months of age so that further cardiopulmonary damage and complications can be prevented.

## Patent ductus arteriosus (PDA)

**Patent ductus arteriosus (PDA)** occurs when the ductus arteriosus that connects the pulmonary artery and aorta fails to close after birth, resulting in left-to-right shunting of blood from the aorta back to the pulmonary artery. This defect increases the blood flow to the lung and causes an increase in pulmonary hypertension that can result in damage to the lung tissue and congestive heart failure. Treatment is initially indomethacin (Indocin), given within 10 days of birth, and this treatment is successful in closing about 80% of defects. However, the other 20% require surgical repair with ligation of the patent vessel. A minimally invasive procedure involves insertion of a coil or other blocking device into the PDA through a catheter. Open surgical repair through a small intercostal incision may be necessary if the catheterization procedure is not successful. Children receive general anesthesia for these procedures.

## Ventricular septal defect

**Ventricular septal defect** is an abnormal opening in the septum between the right and left ventricles. In children, the defect is often congenital; in adults, it may be related to infarction. If the opening is small, the child may be asymptomatic, but larger openings can result in a left-to-right shunt because of higher pressure in the left ventricle. This shunting increases more than 6 weeks after birth, and symptoms become more evident. In some children, the defect may close within a few years, but in others it may persist into adulthood. Symptoms may include signs of congestive heart failure with peripheral edema. About 10% of patients with ventricular septal defect experience Eisenmenger's syndrome, characterized by increased pulmonary hypertension and right-sided heart failure with death often occurring by age 40. Surgical repair includes pulmonary banding or cardiopulmonary bypass repair of the opening with suturing or a patch, depending on the size.

## Lung resection

A number of different procedures are used for **lung resection.** Patients often have lung disease and associated coronary artery and cardiovascular disorders. They commonly have a history of smoking. These factors increase the risk of complications. Numerous factors pose challenges for the anesthetist:

- *Lateral decubitus position:* The dependent lung receives more perfusion and ventilation when the patient is first positioned. During induction, the functional residual capacity decreases, and the dependent lung continues to have better perfusion but decreased ventilation. If controlled positive-pressure ventilation is used, it favors the upper lung, and neuromuscular blocking agents further limit movement of the dependent hemithorax. Proper positioning is necessary for avoiding trauma. The upper arm is extended above the head, and the dependent arm is flexed. The legs are cushioned, and an axillary roll is placed beneath the dependent axilla to prevent injury to the brachial plexus. The dependent eye and ear must be protected from injury and ischemia.

- **Open pneumothorax:** This can lead to hypoxemia and hypercapnia as one lung collapses and a mediastinal shift (toward the dependent lung upon inspiration) and paradoxical respirations occur; therefore, positive-pressure ventilation is necessary.
- **One-lung anesthesia:** A right-to-left intrapulmonary shunt occurs as the collapsed lung is perfused but not ventilated. Oxygenated blood mixes with unoxygenated blood, resulting in hypoxemia. This is counteracted by hypoxic pulmonary vasoconstriction (HPV) (autoregulation mechanism), but this effect is inhibited by extremes of pulmonary artery pressures, hypocapnia, extremes of mixed venous $Po_2$, use of vasodilators, infection, and inhalation anesthetics. Additionally, factors that decrease perfusion of the ventilated lung (high PEEP, hyperventilation), low $Fio_2$, and use of vasoconstrictors may contribute to inhibition of HPV.
- **Monitoring:** Direct arterial pressure and central venous access for CVP measurements are required as part of monitoring. Pulmonary artery catheterization is necessary for some conditions (such as cor pulmonale or left ventricular abnormalities). Transesophageal echocardiography (TEE) monitors cardiac function.

## Lung resection anesthesia

Premedication may be restricted because of lung disease, but anticholinergics may be administered to decrease secretions. Catheters for neuraxial anesthesia or analgesia (for postoperative pain control) may be placed before induction. Preoxygenation is performed before induction with an IV anesthetic agent (often propofol, although ketamine may be used in emergency thoracotomy). Deep anesthesia should be achieved before laryngoscopy to prevent bronchospasm. Anesthesia is usually maintained with a volatile anesthetic agent (halothane, isoflurane, sevoflurane, or desflurane), an opioid, and controlled ventilation. Inhalational anesthetics are used because they depress airway reflexes, are eliminated rapidly, and do not inhibit hypoxic pulmonary constriction, making them particularly useful in maintaining oxygenation with one-lung anesthesia. Nondepolarizing NMBAs are used to facilitate ventilation. Nitrous oxide is avoided or limited to 50% until adequate oxygenation is demonstrated. Hyperinflation of the lungs is used to remove pleural air at the end of the procedure. Extubation is performed upon return of spontaneous ventilation and respiratory reflexes.

## Lung volume reduction

**Lung volume reduction surgery (LVRS)** usually involves removing approximately 20% to 35% of lung tissue that is not functioning adequately. This reduces the size of the lungs so that they work more effectively. This procedure is most commonly used for adult emphysematous COPD patients; these patients are often severely compromised. Patients should stop smoking 6 to 12 weeks before surgery. In adults, surgery is usually bilateral; however, some patients are not candidates for bilateral surgery because of cardiac disease or emphysema affecting only one lung. Unilateral surgery has been shown to be effective. Surgical removal of part of the lung improves ventilation and gas exchange and does not require the immunosuppressive therapy required for lung transplantation. The procedure may be performed through an open-chest thoracotomy or through a less-invasive video-assisted thoracotomy, using one-lung ventilation. Adequate oxygenation and ventilation are essential. The patient should be rapidly extubated so that hyperinflation and barotrauma can be prevented.

## Lobectomy or removing part of the lung tissue

**Lobectomy** removes one or more lobes of a lung (the left lung has 2 lobes; the right lung, 3) and is usually performed for lesions or trauma confined to one lobe, such as tubercular lesions, abscesses or cysts, cancer (usually non-small cell in early stages), traumatic injury, or bronchiectasis. The surgical procedure is usually performed through an open thoracotomy or by video-assisted thoracotomy. Complications can include hemorrhage, postoperative infection with or without abscess formation, and pneumothorax. Usually 1 or 2 chest tubes are left in place in the immediate postsurgical period to remove air, fluid, or both.

**Segmental resection** removes a bronchovascular segment and is used for small lesions in the periphery, bronchiectasis, or congenital cysts or blebs.

**Wedge resection** removes a small wedged-shaped portion of the lung tissue and is used for small peripheral lesions, granulomas, or blebs.

**Bronchoplastic (sleeve) reconstruction** removes part of the bronchus and lung tissue with reanastomosis of the bronchus. This procedure is used for small lesions of the carina or bronchus.

### Pneumonectomy

**Pneumonectomy** is surgical removal of one of the lungs. There are 2 surgical procedures:

- *Simple*: removal of only the lung
- *Extrapleural*: removal of the lung and also part of the diaphragm on the affected side and the pericardium on that same side.

During the operative procedure, much care must be taken to prevent contamination of the remaining lung, including using bronchus blockers or placing the patient in the prone position. Removal of the lung is indicated for a number of conditions, including severe bronchiectasis from chronic suppurative pneumonia, resulting in dilation of terminal bronchioles; severe hypoplasia; unilateral lung destruction with pulmonary hypertension; cancerous lesions; lobar emphysema; chronic pulmonary infection with tissue destruction and hemorrhage. Surgery may be complicated by bronchopleural fistula, empyema, and air leaks. Empyema should be drained preoperatively if possible, and the fistula should be closed. Neuraxial anesthesia or analgesia is often used as an adjunct to general anesthesia for postoperative pain control.

### One-lung anesthesia

**One-lung anesthesia** is frequently used with thoracotomy to prevent contamination or spillage (as from hemorrhage, infection or lavage), to control ventilation, and to allow better surgical access for partial or complete lung resection or transplantation, thoracic aneurysm repair, resection of the esophagus, and anterior procedures on the thoracic spine. ETTs include the following:

- Double-lumen bronchial tubes have two tubes, one entering a bronchus (right or left) and the other remaining in the trachea. The tubes have both bronchial and tracheal cuffs that are inflated to direct air flow to only one lung. Right-bronchus cuffs must have a slit to ventilate the upper lobe, although it is not always adequate because of anatomical differences; therefore, many anesthetists use left-bronchus tubes for both sides. Improper placement of double-lumen tubes is indicated by inadequate lung compliance and decreased exhaled tidal volume. Care must be used to avoid trauma and rupture associated with overinflation. After correct insertion, breath sounds and thorax movement should cease in the nonventilated lung.

- Single-lumen bronchial tubes with bronchial blocker (high-pressure, low-volume cuff) (Univent) require that the blocker be positioned and inflated with a flexible bronchoscope. This tube has an advantage over double-lumen tubes in that it can be used for postoperative intubation, whereas the double-lumen tube must be replaced with an endotracheal tube (ETT). However, the cuff has a small channel that allows the lung to deflate; therefore, deflation occurs slowly and is sometimes incomplete. An alternative procedure uses a regular ETT in conjunction with an inflatable 3-mL Fogarty catheter as a blocker, but this procedure is less stable because the catheter is easily dislodged.
- Single-lumen bronchial tubes (without bronchial blocker) (Gordon-Green) have both bronchial and tracheal cuffs that are inflated or deflated to direct airflow. They are rarely used.

Careful management of respiratory status must be maintained throughout the procedure:

- A high level of fraction of inspired oxygen ($Fio_2$) of 1.0 should be administered to control arterial hypoxemia.
- Tidal ventilation of the dependent lung is initiated at 8 to 10 mL/kg because lower volumes may result in atelectasis.
- Minute ventilation must be maintained at the same level as with bilateral ventilation; therefore, the rate must be adjusted accordingly.
- $Paco_2$ should be about 40 mm Hg, similar to that used for bilateral ventilation.
- Oxygen saturation must be continually monitored, and arterial blood gases must be measured after approximately 15 minutes of one-lung ventilation.
- Hypoxemia must be immediately controlled through repositioning of tube, reinflating the non-dependent lung, and using continuous positive airway pressure (CPAP) to increase oxygen transport.
- Positive end-expiratory pressure (PEEP) is used at 5 to 10 cm $H_2O$ for the dependent lung.
- Patient is repositioned if necessary.
- Bilateral ventilation is resumed if necessary.

## Thymectomy

The **thymus** is located substernally and is part of the body's immune system, aiding in lymphocyte maturation into T cells. Tumors may arise from epithelial cells of the thymus, forming thymomas. These occur in 25% to 50% of patients with myasthenia gravis and are usually benign; however, the thymus exhibits abnormal lymphoid hyperplasia in myasthenia patients. Researchers believe that this abnormal tissue may cause an autoimmune response affecting the neuromuscular system. **Thymectomy** is performed to relieve symptoms; it effects improvement or remission of symptoms for approximately 70% of patients who undergo the procedure. The surgical procedure may be performed with a transcervical or transsternal approach. Patients often receive combined general and neuraxial anesthesia to provide postoperative pain relief and to facilitate early extubation. Postoperative respiratory failure can result from exacerbations of symptoms or muscle relaxants. A newer minimally invasive technique, robotic thoracoscopic thymectomy (*da Vinci*), requires only 3 small incisions in the left chest and uses robotic arms to excise the thymus.

### Intrathoracic surgical procedures required for hiatal hernias

A **hiatal hernia** is a defect in the diaphragm. The opening (hiatus) through which the esophagus passes enlarges, allowing the stomach to herniate into the chest and causing damage to the esophagus. Types of hiatal hernias include the following:

- *Type I – Sliding (90%):* Both the stomach and the gastroesophageal junction herniate upward and slide in and out of the thorax. This type of hernia is associated with reflux because damage occurs to the gastroesophageal sphincter.
- *Types II-IV – Paraesophageal:* All or part of the stomach herniates through the opening beside the esophageal junction and the esophagus. This type of hernia is not associated with reflux. Paraesophageal hernias may rotate, restricting blood flow and requiring emergency surgery.

Surgical repair with general anesthesia may be performed through an abdominal incision with the hiatus tightened and sometimes with a fundoplication to tighten the sphincter. A laparoscopic procedure may be possible. An endoluminal fundoplication is a minimally invasive procedure using an endoscope to place clips about the esophagus to tighten the sphincter.

### Diaphragmatic hernias or ruptures

**Acquired diaphragmatic hernia** involves herniation of abdominal contents into the chest cavity; it is usually caused by trauma (blunt or penetrating) from motor vehicle accidents, gunshot wounds, or stabbing. Diaphragmatic hernia or rupture may also be caused by labor or by barotrauma associated with underwater diving. Left-sided rupture is more common because the right diaphragm is stronger. Patients with pronounced hernias or rupture usually have profound dyspnea, bowel sounds in the chest, severe abdominal pain, and paradoxical abdominal breathing patterns. Surgical repair is always necessary, even for minor hernias, to prevent strangulation. If related to acute trauma, repair may be with laparoscopy or thoracotomy, depending on the extent of injury. An abdominal approach may be used if other abdominal injuries are suspected. Latent hernias may require a transthoracic approach because of adhesions. General anesthesia with positive-pressure ventilation is often used.

### Esophagectomy

Many surgical approaches to **esophagectomy** may be used.

- *Transhiatal* approach requires an upper abdominal and left cervical incision. Retractors may compromise cardiac function; manipulation may block cardiac filling, causing hypotension; and vagal stimulation may occur.
- *En bloc thoracic* approach requires posterior thoracotomy, abdominal incision, and left cervical incision, and this involves changes in the patient's position. This procedure is often used for adenocarcinoma after neoadjuvant therapy. In some cases, the thoracic portion of the procedure is performed by thoracoscopy, which results in less respiratory depression.
- *Colonic interposition* approach (pedicle graft of the colon) requires an extended surgical procedure and fluid shifts; therefore, maintaining hemodynamic status may be difficult. Because perfusion is crucial if the graft is to survive, BP, cardiac output, and hemoglobin concentration must be monitored and maintained at adequate levels.
- *Gastric pull-up* approach requires that the stomach be literally pulled up and anastomosed to the cervical esophagus. This procedure is often performed with the patient under both general and thoracic epidural anesthesia.

## Esophagus intrathoracic surgical procedures

Surgery of the **esophagus** is performed to remove tumors (usually squamous cell carcinomas or adenocarcinomas) or to treat gastroesophageal reflux or achalasia. All procedures pose a similar risk of aspiration, especially with obstruction or impaired sphincter. Surgery is usually performed with the patient in the supine head-up position and uses rapid-sequence induction with cricoid pressure and general anesthesia. Metoclopramide or proton-pump inhibitors may be given preoperatively to reduce the risk of aspiration, and extubation should be performed after emergence. Fiberoptic intubation may be used in some conditions, such as scleroderma, to avoid trauma. A double-lumen tube may be used for thoracotomy or thoracoscopy. If dilation of the esophagus is indicated, an esophageal bougie may be used (with care to avoid trauma). Some procedures, such as esophagectomy, involve considerable blood loss and require invasive monitoring throughout the procedures, including monitoring of arterial and central venous pressure.

## Surgical procedures of the neck

### Pharyngectomy, laryngectomy, and radical neck resection

**Pharyngectomy and laryngectomy** may be performed as part of a **radical neck resection** for cancer of the throat. The procedure may be extensive and may include the tongue, parotid glands, and part of the mandible. Therefore, the extent of the procedure varies according to the lesion. In some cases, tracheostomy may be needed, and some reconstructive procedures, such as a flap, may be performed at the time of the initial procedure. Most patients are elderly and have comorbid conditions related to alcohol and tobacco use. Some have had radiotherapy before surgery; therefore, managing the airway can pose a challenge to the anesthetist. IV induction is avoided in favor of inhalational induction when the airway is compromised. Tracheostomy equipment should be available during intubation, especially if the lesion may be dislodged. Invasive monitoring is usually indicated so that blood pressure, blood gas, and hematocrit (to evaluate blood loss) can be measured. At least two IV lines should be in place but should not be placed in a limb used for a donor flap.

Gases should be heated and warming blankets should be used to prevent hypothermia, which can interfere with perfusion of flap. The tracheostomy is often performed during laryngectomy, which increases the risk of aspiration and decreased ventilation. Incorrect positioning of the tube or tracheal obstruction due to debris may be indicated by increased peak inspiratory pressure after the tube is inserted. In some cases, neuromuscular blocking agents may be omitted so that nerve function can be assessed. There is danger of decreased cerebral perfusion if the procedure involves the carotid artery or the jugular vein, and danger of venous air embolism if the head must be raised. Vasoconstrictors and vasodilators should be avoided, although there may be considerable hypotensive or hypertensive episodes and cardiac abnormalities because of manipulation of the stellate ganglion and the carotid sinus. The carotid sheath may be infiltrated with local anesthetic to control these problems.

## Laryngeal fractures

**Laryngeal fractures** most often result from severe trauma, such as motor vehicle accident. There are a number of possible fractures or dislocations:

- *Cricoarytenoid joint:* Dislocation cause by compression of the larynx against a cervical vertebra.
- *Cricothyroid joint:* Displacement of the thyroid cartilage behind the cricoid cartilage may injure the laryngeal nerve and cause paralysis of vocal cords.
- *Glottis:* Fractures of thyroid cartilage near vocal cords.
- *Hyoid:* Usually medial; most occur in women.
- *Subglottis*: Injury of cricothyroid joint resulting in damage to laryngeal nerve and paralysis of vocal cords (bilaterally).
- *Supraglottis*: Horizontal fractures with displacement of epiglottis.

Laryngeal injuries are often associated with intracranial or cervical injuries; therefore, the airway must always be carefully examined, especially with cervical injuries and in the presence of indications of dyspnea, hoarseness or difficulty speaking, difficulty swallowing, subcutaneous emphysema, or neck pain. If the airway is compromised, immediate tracheostomy, direct laryngoscopy, esophagoscopy, or explorative surgery may be indicated.

## Parathyroid glands

The **parathyroid glands** (usually 4) are located behind the thyroid gland. They produce parathormone (PTH), which regulates calcium and phosphorus metabolism. Most symptoms of hyperthyroidism relate to hypercalcemia. If a single adenoma exists, then surgery excision of only that lesion may be possible; however, if there is hyperplasia, all 4 parathyroid glands are usually removed. There are a number of problems related to general anesthesia:

- Increased calcium levels may cause hypertension and arrhythmias; therefore, calcium concentration should be normalized (<14 mg/dL) with normal saline (NS) and furosemide or bisphosphonates.
- Hypoventilation may cause acidosis and increase ionized calcium levels.
- Hyperventilation may cause alkalosis and decrease ionized calcium levels.
- Response to neuromuscular blocking agents may be impaired.
- Vertebral osteoporosis due to leaching of calcium may predispose to cervical compression or fractures during laryngoscopy.
- Blood products with citrate must be administered slowly to avoid decreased calcium concentrations.

## Thyroid

**Hyperthyroidism** (thyrotoxicosis) usually results from excessive production of thyroid hormones (Graves' disease) caused by abnormal stimulation from immunoglobulins. Other causes include thyroiditis and excessive thyroid medications. Symptoms vary and include anxiety, tachycardia, atrial fibrillation, tremor, exophthalmos, and progressive weakness. The thyroid is surgically removed if patients cannot tolerate other treatments or in special circumstances, such as large goiter. Usually one-sixth of the thyroid is left in place and antithyroid medications are given before the procedure. Preoperative medication includes benzodiazepines. The surgical procedure is performed with the patient under general anesthesia and IV induction agents, such as thiopental. Incision is at base of the throat. A nondepolarizing NMBA may facilitate intubation of patients with

- 60 -

an enlarged goiter. Maintenance is usually with a volatile anesthetic (isoflurane), which blunts sympathetic responses. Temperature and ECG must be monitored to observe for onset of thyroid storm. Cooling blankets must be available in case temperature rises. Hypotension is usually treated with phenylephrine. A continuous lumbar epidural anesthetic (without epinephrine) may be used to blockade the sympathetic nervous system.

## Cervical spine

Surgical approaches to relieving pain and disability related to herniated disks include the following: discectomy alone or with spinal fusion; partial, half, or complete laminectomy; and foraminotomy. The **cervical spine** is particularly vulnerable to stress, and most lesions occur at the C5-C6 and C6-C7 interspaces. Injury may cause stiffness, pain, and paresthesia of upper extremities. Discectomy with or without fusion may be required to provide relief of symptoms. Neurological monitoring during surgery is important because ischemia to the spinal cord can cause neurological impairment. Blood is supplied by the anterior spinal artery (ASA), which supplies the anterior two-thirds of the spinal cord, and by two posterior spinal arteries (PSAs), which supply the posterior one-third. Impaired perfusion through the ASA can cause motor deficit and loss of sensations to pain and temperature. (Additional blood flow is supplied by radicular arteries to the lower spinal cord. These anastomose to the ASA and PSAs.)

## Cervical spine repair (anterior and posterior approaches)

- *Anterior approach*: The patient receives general anesthesia while in the supine position with the neck hyperextended. A transverse incision is made, usually on the left side of the neck (a right-sided approach poses greater risk of injuring nerves). The tissue is separated, and retractors hold the wound open so that the surgeon can access the anterior spine to remove the disk with or without fusion. Complications include airway obstruction; carotid, thyroid, or vertebral artery injury; injury to laryngeal or phrenic nerves; perforation of the esophagus; and dural tears.
- *Posterior approach*: This approach is usually used for fusion of cervical fractures, dislocations, or deformities, such as kyphosis. The patient receives general anesthesia and is placed in the prone position with the head anchored. A midline incision is made in the cervical area to allow access to the posterior spine. Complications include damage to the nerve root, which can result in muscle weakness.

## Forcervical spine

Blood flow to the spinal cord is about 40% of the blood flow to the brain. The thoracic area receives half of the blood flow received by the cervical and lumbar areas; therefore, the thoracic region of the spine is most vulnerable to ischemic injury. Somatosensory evoked potentials (SSEP) have been used for neurological monitoring, but studies show that they may miss injury during cervical approaches. Myogenic transcranial motor-evoked potentials (MEPs) are more accurate, but they are incompatible with some anesthetic agents: volatile anesthetics, neuromuscular blockade with loss of more than 2 twitches in train of 4, nitrous oxide >50%, and thiopental and midazolam as induction agents. Thus, with MEP monitoring, general anesthesia is usually totally intravenous. If the patient has severe limitations in cervical mobility, intubation while the patient is awake may be necessary.

## Lymph node biopsy

The **lymph nodes** in the neck are a drainage site for metastatic malignant oral lesions. Therefore, when an oropharyngeal lesion is found or a neck mass is evident, a biopsy of lymph nodes in the neck is indicated, because positive findings help identify the type of tumor by its source:

- Postauricular and posterior triangle: Nasopharyngeal, scalp, ear, and skull-base malignancies.
- Submandibular: Oral malignancies.
- Submental: Lip malignancies.
- Supraclavicular: Thyroid or esophageal malignancies.
- Deep lateral cervical: Oral malignancies.

Biopsy may be performed to determine the cause of enlarged lymph nodes, to aid in diagnosis, and to stage a cancerous lesion to determine whether it has metastasized. Biopsy is usually performed with the patient under local anesthesia and in the supine position with the neck hyperextended. Several types of biopsy are possible: fine-needle aspiration, core biopsy, and incisional biopsy.

## Tracheal repair

**Tracheal repair** is rare but is necessary for a variety of conditions: congenital stenosis, complete tracheal rings, postintubation stenosis, trauma, cancer, and tracheomalacia. A variety of procedures are used for repair, depending on the extent of involvement and other concomitant anomalies, such as pulmonary artery sling or bronchial abnormalities. Premedication is avoided with airway obstruction. Inhalation induction with 100% oxygen should be slow, and NMBAs should be avoided. IV lidocaine may be used to deepen anesthesia for laryngoscopy. A bronchoscopy may be performed, and the patient can then be intubated with a small tube that can avoid the obstruction. The type of incision relates to the lesion; a collar incision used for high lesions. As the trachea is bisected, the surgeon places an armored tube in the distal portion, and the anesthetist connects this tube to ventilation. After reanastomosis, the armored tube is withdrawn and the original intubation tube is again used. Lesions in the lower trachea may require more-complicated procedures with sternotomy, thoracotomy, or cardiopulmonary bypass (CPB) and high-frequency ventilation.

<u>Tracheal repair (resection and anastomosis, slide tracheoplasty, pericardial patch, and autologous graft)</u>
Procedures for **tracheal repair**:

- *Resection and anastomosis* is effective if less than 30% of the trachea is involved; therefore, this procedure is used for short-segment stenosis.
- *Slide tracheoplasty* involves transecting the stenotic area and spatulating (making longitudinal cuts above and below the transection and then spreading the tissue to enlarge it) before reanastomosis. Slide tracheoplasty is used for long-segment stenosis with excellent results. This procedure uses the patient's own tissue, but follow-up bronchoscopies are necessary to remove the granulation tissue that tends to form.
- *Pericardial patch* repairs the trachea by creating an autologous graft from a section of the pericardium. This procedure provides a good graft and rapid healing but requires cardiopulmonary bypass.
- *Autologous graft* may be created by using excised stenotic tracheal tissue for an anterior patch.

<u>Tracheal repair (intraluminal stents)</u>

- ***Intraluminal stents*** may be used to support and prepare the trachea for further repair or to repair a failed tracheoplasty. A variety of stents are used, including the Dumon silastic stent, which provides good support and is easily removed but cannot provide dilation. The metallic Palmaz stent is balloon-expandable and can be used to dilate a stenotic trachea, but it can be difficult to remove if granulation tissue grows through the meshwork of the stent. This problem can be managed with repeated balloon dilations to provide pressure against the granulation tissue. Wire stents are permanent but require periodic dilation.

In some cases, ventilation must be continued after the surgical procedure to ensure adequate airflow, but the goal of anesthesia is to extubate the patient as soon as possible to prevent the ETT from causing damage, such as tissue necrosis.

**Tracheotomy (percutaneous thyrotomy)**

The trachea ("windpipe") is part of the airway that extends from C6 to T5 and is approximately 10 to 15 cm long. It is supported by 16 to 20 semicircular cartilages. The cricoid cartilage (at the top) forms a complete circle. **Tracheotomy,** a surgically created tracheal opening, creates a temporary or permanent tracheostomy to provide an airway and to use for mechanical ventilation (especially for ventilation for more than 7 days). Patients are positioned with the neck supported and hyperextended (if possible). Patients are preoxygenated and are usually premedicated with a combination of benzodiazepine (midazolam), an opioid (such as morphine), and an NMBA. The patient receives local anesthesia and IV anesthesia and is intubated. During the procedure, the ETT must be partially withdrawn as the incision is made. There are a number of procedures:

- ***Percutaneous thyrotomy*** may be performed in emergency situations with a 14-guage IV catheter (not recommended for children younger than 10 years) immediately above the cricoid cartilage in the cricothyroid membrane. This thyrotomy may later be replaced by a surgical tracheostomy.
- ***Standard tracheotomy:*** An incision is made into the trachea, and pretracheal tissue is completely excised. A tracheostomy tube is inserted into the opening to provide a conduit and maintain the opening.
- **Minimally invasive percutaneous tracheotomy** (PCT) comprises a number of newer techniques (not recommended for children younger than 15) that are performed surgically but are less traumatic. All of these techniques use a guide wire and special kits to dilate and prepare an opening for a tracheostomy tube. Needles or tubes are inserted between the first and second or the second and third rings for all procedures:
- ***Guidewire dilating forceps (GWDF):*** A small incision is made below the cricoid cartilage. An IV needle (14 gauge) is inserted, and the needle is removed and the cannula advanced. A guidewire (Seldinger) is inserted through the cannula and the cannula is removed. Special forceps are inserted into the opening and then opened to dilate the opening. A tracheostomy tube is passed over the wire, and the wire is then removed.
- ***Percutaneous dilational tracheostomy (PDT):*** Small (1.5- to 2-cm) incisions are made at the first and second cartilage ring with a blunt midline dissection. A needle (22 gauge) is inserted and, when the needle has been positioned, a guidewire is passed through the needle. A series of dilators are passed over the guidewire to enlarge the opening. The tracheostomy tube is passed over the dilator and guidewire and is positioned; the guidewire and dilator are then removed, leaving the tube in place.

- ***Rapitrach:*** Incision is made as with other procedures. Blunt dissection of subcutaneous tissue is done by forceps until tracheal rings are palpable. A needle (12 gauge) is inserted, a guidewire passed, and the needle removed. A special dilator tool is passed over the guidewire and opened to dilate the stoma, and then the tracheostomy tube is inserted through the open dilator. The guidewire and dilator are removed.

### Neuroskeletal surgical procedures: laminectomy

**Laminectomy** is commonly performed to relieve symptoms of spinal stenosis, in which a disc collapses, encroaching on the spinal canal and compressing nerves. The posterior longitudinal ligament pushes inward as the space between vertebrae narrows, and bone spurs may grow into the canal. Normally, the spinal canal has a circumference of 1.7 to 1.8 cm, but this circumference can shrink to 1.0 cm with stenosis related to congenital defects, disk herniation, and instability from stretched or damaged ligaments and tendons, or degeneration from back injury or bone spurs. Laminectomy removes part or all of the lamina, bone spurs, and ligaments to relieve pressure on the nerves or to allow access to the spine for other surgical procedures, such as removal of tumors. Laminectomy may be combined with discectomy. Laminectomy can be performed at any level of the vertebrae. Cervical and thoracic laminectomies pose the greatest danger of paralysis from nerve damage. Laminectomy is performed with the patient under general anesthesia, usually with the patient in the prone kneeling position.

The standard laminectomy is much more invasive than newer microscopic and percutaneous procedures and requires a much longer recovery period:

- ***Standard laminectomy:*** This involves dissection of muscle tissue and removal of all or part of the lamina and the spinal processes, as well as connective tissue and tendons. The posterior spinal ligament may be excised to allow access to the nerve root for decompression. This procedure lasts for 1 to 3 hours and requires the use of general anesthesia.
- ***Minimally invasive (microendoscopic) laminectomy***: Typically, a needle is inserted into the surgical area and a small (approximately 2 cm) incision is made. Dilators or instruments are inserted to push aside the muscles and ligaments to allow access and passage of a hollow tube, through which a microscopic endoscope is passed. Fiberoptics allow video images to be viewed on a monitor. Microscopic tools cut away tissue and bone to decompress the nerve. This procedure can be performed with the patient under general or spinal anesthesia. This procedure usually lasts for approximately 15 minutes.

### Neuroskeletal surgical procedures: fusion

**Spinal fusion** is performed to correct abnormal curvatures (such as with kyphosis or scoliosis), unstable vertebrae (often after removal of tumors), and herniated discs. It is being increasingly used to treat low back pain. With a spinal fusion, 2 or more vertebrae are essentially fused. In some cases, the disk is removed. A bone graft is typically used to fill the space between vertebrae. This may be an autogenous graft, often from the pelvic bone, or an allograft graft from a donor. Sometimes, stabilizing materials, such as rods, screws, and plates, are used to secure the vertebrae. This procedure is usually performed with the patient under general anesthesia in the spinal lordosis position (for lumbar fusions), and incisions may be performed through the back or through the abdomen (for the lumbar region). Newer minimally invasive procedures with a microscopic endoscope may be performed through the abdomen (4 small incisions), the back (one small incision), or the flank, depending on the type of fusion, anterior or posterior.

# Neuroskeletal surgical procedures required for the spinal cord

Patients with acute **spinal cord injuries** should immediately be evaluated for airway control; the spine should be immobilized. Most injuries result from trauma and vertebral fractures or dislocations that cause partial or complete transection of the spinal cord. Transection is most common at C5-C6 and T12-L1. In some cases, symptoms are reversible if surgical decompression is performed immediately. Unstable spinal columns also require immediate repair. Treatment includes the following:

- Intubation and ventilation (usually with sedation) to prevent respiratory failure for injuries at C5 or above.
- Intravenous fluids to prevent and treat hypotension.
- Corticosteroids for neurological deficits from blunt trauma:
- Begin within 8 hours of injury.
- Methylprednisolone 30 mg/kg bolus IV over 15 minutes.
- 45-minute break.
- Methylprednisolone 5.4 mg/kg per hour for 23 hours.
- Surgical decompression as needed, depending on the site and degree of injury, or spinal stabilization. A combination of the two techniques may also be used.

Direct arterial, CV, and pulmonary artery pressure monitoring is necessary.

Both hypotension and bradycardia may be present before induction; therefore, general anesthesia may be administered with IV bolus and ketamine. Succinylcholine should not be used for more than 24 hours because it may cause hyperkalemia. Patients with ***chronic spinal cord injuries*** pose different problems, because those with injuries above T6 may develop autonomic hyperreflexia with surgical manipulation. A combination of general anesthesia with volatile anesthetics and neuraxial anesthesia should be used to prevent hyperreflexia; however, neuraxial anesthesia can be difficult to administer because of previous injury and deformities, the potential for increasing hypotension, and difficulty in determining the degree of anesthesia. Nitroprusside may be necessary to control hyperreflexia. Nondepolarizing NMBAs are usually used rather than succinylcholine to reduce the danger of hyperkalemia (although this rarely occurs after 6 months). Body temperature is monitored because patients may have chronic vasodilation that predisposes them to hypothermia. Agents primarily excreted through the kidneys should be avoided.

# Neuroskeletal surgical procedures: surgical sympathectomy

**Surgical sympathectomy** is destruction of nerves of the sympathetic system, either by cutting, cauterizing, or clipping, for the purpose of decreasing pain, increasing blood flow, or reducing anhidrosis. The procedure is used specifically for Raynaud's disease, claudication (lower extremities), excessive sweating, and reflex sympathetic dystrophy. Before sympathectomy, a temporary ganglion block may be performed with steroids or local anesthetic to evaluate response. The traditional approach requires general anesthesia and a midspinal vertical incision, but sympathectomy is now usually performed by using minimally invasive techniques with the patient under local anesthesia. For anhidrosis, a small subaxillary incision is made with insufflation of the thoracic cavity and introduction of a fiberoptic endoscope to locate the nerve, which is cut with microscopic instruments. In some cases, percutaneous radiofrequency ablation may be used. The nerve is isolated through by radiography electrical stimulation; radio waves are then directed at it through electrodes. Sympathectomy is successful in relieving symptoms in 75% to 90% of patients.

## Neuroskeletal surgical procedures: vertebroplasty

**Vertebroplasty** is a minimally invasive technique for treating compression fractures. It may be used for chronic pain related to osteoporotic compression fractures or to relieve acute pain. Typically, the procedure is performed with the patient in the prone position and with conscious sedation (such as midazolam) and local anesthetic. Under image guidance, a large-bore needle (trocar) is inserted through a tiny nick and through the spinal muscles into holes in weakened vertebrae. Osseous venography may be performed to determine correct placement of the needle. Bone cement, polymethylmethacrylate (PMMA), is injected into the bone to stabilize it. Once injected, the cement sets in approximately 15 minutes. Multiple injections may be needed, depending on the extent of injury and the number of vertebrae treated. Often, pain relief is immediate, and most patients experience relief within 48 hours. A CT scan may be used upon completion of the vertebroplasty to verify the cement distribution. No suturing is necessary.

## Vascular surgical procedures: carotid

Carotid stenosis usually results from atherosclerosis; therefore, patients are at increased risk of coronary artery and peripheral vascular disease. **Carotid endarterectomy** (CAE) involves cross-clamping the carotid and then opening and removing the plaque that is occluding the artery. A shunt may be inserted during the procedure to ensure blood supply to the brain. Traditionally, CAE was performed with the patient under general anesthesia, but the use of regional anesthesia (deep and superficial cervical nerve blocks) and awake sedation allows for better monitoring of cerebral function. With general anesthesia, indirect monitoring may be performed with bispectral index, jugular venous oxygen saturation, stump bleeding and pressure, EEG, and evoked potentials. Intraoperative complications include the following:

- Bradycardia because of vagus nerve stimulation.
- Tachycardia caused by catecholamine release with manipulation of the carotid sinus. Hypotension from anesthetic agents and from unclamping the carotid.
- Hypertension with sympathetic stimulation.

Because of the lability of BP and cardiovascular status, IV lines with nitroprusside and neo-synephrine should be available so that the medications can be administered rapidly.

## Thoracic aorta

Surgical repair of the **descending thoracic aorta** (distal, Stanford type B, DeBakey type III) is either through a left thoracotomy or a thoracoabdominal incision (depending on location of lesion) without cardiopulmonary bypass (CPB). One-lung anesthesia may be used to facilitate access. Invasive monitoring should include arterial blood pressure via the right radial artery, pulmonary artery catheterization, and transesophageal echocardiography (TEE). Because intraoperative bleeding may be pronounced, a cell-saver is often used for autotransfusion. Cross-clamping of the aorta causes hypertension above the clamp, which may cause left ventricular failure and myocardial ischemia. Nitroprusside is usually administered to prevent hypertension and decreased cardiac output, although it must be used carefully because hypotension may increase the danger of spinal cord injury due to ischemia. Hypotension occurs below the clamp. This may also cause ischemia of the spinal cord and paraplegia, especially if the aorta is clamped for longer than 30 minutes.

Distal perfusion may be improved by the use of a heparin-coated shunt or partial CPB with hypothermia, although CPB requires heparinization, which may increase bleeding. Methylprednisolone and mannitol may be used to prevent spinal ischemia by decreasing CSF pressure. In some cases, CSF is drained via a catheter to reduce pressure. Mannitol is often infused before cross-clamping, especially for patients with renal disease, to prevent renal failure, which may occur after surgery. Releasing the cross-clamp can cause intravascular instability because it this can cause severe hypotension when vasodilating metabolites from the ischemic areas of the body are released. Slow release coupled with decreased anesthetic depth and volume loading may prevent excessive hypotension. Metabolic acidosis must be monitored and may be treated with sodium bicarbonate. Most patients remain intubated with mechanical ventilation for 2 to 24 hours after surgery.

## Abdominal aorta surgical procedures

**Abdominal aorta** repair is the most common and is usually done for large (> 5cm) or dissecting aortic aneurysm. The procedure is usually performed with an anterior transperitoneal or an anterolateral retroperitoneal approach. This procedure requires heparinization before cross-clamping at the supraceliac, suprarenal, or infrarenal (causes least hemodynamic changes on clamping) aorta. Complications are similar to those associated with thoracic aorta repair, especially hypotension related to release of the cross clamp. Fluid requirements are usually large and require the IV administration of combination colloid and crystalloid at 10 to 12 mL/kg/hr in addition to fluid replacement for blood loss. Monitoring includes intraarterial blood pressure (either side), central venous or pulmonary artery pressure, and TEE. Mannitol is used as a prophylaxis, especially for patients with renal disease and those undergoing clamping of the infrarenal aorta. A combination of general and epidural anesthesia may be used to suppress levels of stress hormones and to provide postoperative pain control. However, because the risk of bleeding is increased, a catheter should be placed before heparinization and removed when the results of coagulation studies are stable.

## Arteriovenous graft

An **arteriovenous graft** is a surgically created vascular access. An arteriovenous fistula is the preferred type of vascular access for long-term hemodialysis. The fistula is created by surgically connecting an artery and a vein, most commonly the radial artery and the cephalic vein (Brescia-Comino forearm fistula), although the brachial artery and cephalic vein may also be used. A graft (autogenous, semibiologic, or synthetic) is used to create the fistula. Because the venous portion dilates and hypertrophies over time, it can be used for repeated treatments. The surgical procedure is often performed with the patient under local anesthetic and regional block. Typically, a small (3 cm) lengthwise incision is made between the radial artery and the cephalic vein, and the cephalic vein is loosened and anastomosed to the radial artery. Both systemic and local infusion of heparin is used to prevent clotting. A thrill is felt along the proximal vein after anastomosis unless there is obstruction, which may require further procedures. Prosthetic access (forearm loop or brachioaxillary) grafts are usually inserted with regional anesthesia but may require general anesthesia.

## Peripheral arterial insufficiency surgical procedures

Surgical intravenation for **peripheral arterial insufficiency** and ulcers may be necessary if the response to medical treatment is insufficient, if the pain is intolerable, or if a limb-threatening ischemia or gangrene occurs. Surgical and vascular interventions include the following:

- *Bypass grafts* in which a section of the saphenous vein or an upper extremity vein are harvested and are used to bypass damaged arteries and to supply blood to distal vessels in the leg. Because veins have valves, they must be reversed or stripped of valves before attachment. Synthetic grafts are also sometimes used, but they have a much higher failure rate.
- *Angioplasty* can be performed if disease is not extensive (*extensive* is defined as >10 in length), but arteries must be large enough to safely accommodate the procedure. Initial results are good, but long-term rates have been less positive, although the use of anticoagulants improves success rates.

Surgical procedures may be performed with the patient under general or regional anesthesia, depending on the extent of the procedure. Arteriography, ultrasonography, or both may be performed during surgery.

## Transjugular intrahepatic portosystemic shunt

**Transjugular intrahepatic portosystemic shunt** is a minimally invasive procedure that places a stent within the liver to improve hepatic blood circulation for patients with portal hypertension. The patient is placed in the supine position and receives either IV sedation and local anesthesia or general anesthesia while blood pressure, respiratory status, and cardiac status are monitored. A small nick is made in the skin, and (with ultrasound guidance) a catheter is fed into the jugular vein and (with fluoroscopic guidance) advanced to the liver and into a hepatic vein. Contrast dye may be injected IV to assist with stent placement. The catheter is positioned and a needle is inserted through the catheter to create a channel for the wire-mesh stent (Gore-Tex), which is placed over a balloon-tipped catheter and fed through the original catheter. When the stent is properly positioned, the balloon is inflated, opening the stent. The balloon is deflated and the catheters are removed, leaving the stent to connect the portal vein to the hepatic vein, thereby allowing blood to flow through the liver.

## Renovascular disorders

**Renovascular disorders** occur when blood flow through the renal arteries and veins is impaired by stenosis (usually atherosclerotic). This stenosis increases blood pressure and leads to renal failure or thrombosis (rare), which may dislodge and cause pulmonary embolism. Thrombosis is usually related to nephrotic syndrome, tumors, or infection. Minimally invasive procedures are usually performed with the patient under IV sedation and local anesthesia; more-invasive procedures require general anesthesia. Surgical procedures include the following:

- *Thrombolysis*: A thrombolytic agent is injected into a clot in the renal artery via a catheter, usually during angiography.
- *Angioplasty with stent,* an endovascular procedure, uses a balloon-tip catheter fed into the renal artery to open the vessel and may include placement of a metal-mesh stent through the catheter and into the renal artery to improve renal blood flow.

- **Surgical endarterectomy** removes the inner lining of the renal artery to eliminate plaque.
- **Surgical bypass** uses an endogenous vein graft or synthetic graft to attach to one of the veins and bypass a blocked area.

## Aortic stents

**Endovascular aortic stents** are inserted by means of a minimally invasive procedure while the patient receives IV sedation and a regional or local anesthetic or (in some cases) general anesthesia. A small femoral incision is made, and a guidewire (with fluoroscopic guidance) is advanced to the site of the aneurysm. A catheter is then passed, and angiography is performed with contrast dye to ensure proper placement. The compressed stent (a synthetic fabric [Gore-Tex] tube with wire mesh) is inserted on a sheath (catheter), the stent is opened, and the sheath is removed. The stent expands against the walls of the aorta. More than one graft component may be placed in a similar manner, depending on the degree of injury to the aorta. Complications include endoleaks (between graft components), migration of grafts, infection, and occlusion of graft. Patients must be carefully monitored. Endoleaks can occur postoperatively and as long as years after the procedure, so patients must undergo long-term follow-up.

## Vena cava filters

**Vena cava filters** are small metal net-like devices that are placed into the vena cava to prevent emboli from reaching the lungs. They are used for patients with deep vein thrombosis or those at risk of emboli, such as patients with myocardial infarction, those who have suffered traumatic injuries, or those undergoing complete hip replacement. The filters are often used for those who cannot take anticoagulation therapy or those who have bleeding or serious complications associated with anticoagulation therapy. The procedure is usually performed with the patient under IV sedation and local anesthesia or, in some cases, general anesthesia. The filter is placed by means of a minimally invasive endovascular procedure through a small incision at the jugular or femoral vein. The filter is advanced to the vena cava with a catheter and an insertion device. The filter is placed, and the catheter is removed. Careful monitoring is necessary. Complications include bleeding, stroke, and pulmonary embolism. Heparin may be used during the procedure to reduce clotting.

## Diagnostic/therapeutic procedures

### Arterial catheterization (radial)

**Arterial catheterization** is routinely performed to monitor arterial blood pressure. Various sites may be used (ulnar, femoral, brachial, dorsalis pedia and posterior tibial, axillary) but the radial artery is most commonly used because of adequate collateral blood flow and ease of insertion. Similar techniques are used for all sites. Insertion may be performed after the patient has been sedated. A local anesthetic (lidocaine) is injected above the artery after it has been located by palpation. An 18-gauge needle is typically used to puncture the skin; an 18- to 22-gauge needle with a catheter is then inserted at a 45° angle. When blood flashback indicates proper placement, the needle angle is decreased to 30° and the needle is advanced 1 to 2 mm so that the tip of the catheter is inside the lumen. The catheter is advanced and the needle is removed, and the catheter is attached to a catheter-tubing transducer system leading to a monitor. The catheter is secured with tape or a suture.

### Pulmonary artery catheterization

**Pulmonary artery catheterization (PAC)** is indicated for cardiac disease; respiratory disease; fluid management in complex cases, such as trauma, shock and burns; high-risk surgical

- 69 -

procedures; and high-risk obstetric complications (toxemia, placentae abruptio). Typical catheters have 5 lumens:

- Wiring to connect the thermistor to a thermodilution cardiac output computer.
- Balloon inflation channel.
- Proximal port for infusions, cardiac output injections, and measurement of right atrial pressure
- Ventricular port for drug infusion.
- Distal port to provide access for mixed venous blood samples (partial pressure of mixed venous oxygen $Pvo_2$ is normally 40 mm Hg with 75% saturation) and pulmonary artery pressure measurement

The catheter is inserted into the right internal jugular vein with the patient in the Trendelenburg position as for central venous catheterization. The catheter's balloon must be checked, and the lumens must be irrigated with heparinized saline before to insertion. Usually, an 18-gauge needle is used to access the vein and a J-wire (guidewire) is inserted through the needle. A dilator and a sheath are then threaded over the J-wire.

## Pulmonary artery catheterization

The dilator and J-wire are removed, and the PAC is threaded through the sheath and the internal jugular vein. It reaches the right atrium at about 15 cm. The balloon is inflated (usually 1.5 mL) to prevent the catheter tip from causing trauma and to allow pressure from the right ventricular cardiac output to float the catheter upward into the pulmonary artery as it is advanced. In difficult cases, flotation may be facilitated by raising the patient's head, asking the patient to inhale deeply, or administering an inotropic agent to increase cardiac output. Iced saline may stiffen the catheter and make insertion easier, but this stiffness increases the danger of perforation. Constant ECG monitoring is necessary to ensure proper placement:

- Increased systolic pressure on distal tracing indicates right ventricular placement.
- Increased diastolic pressure indicates pulmonary artery placement.

Chest radiography is used to verify position. Many complications can occur: bleeding, pneumothorax, air embolism, dysrhythmias, heart block, pulmonary artery rupture, thrombophlebitis, thrombus, endocarditis, sepsis, and death.

## Central venous catheterization

**Central venous catheterization** is performed to monitor intravascular volume and cardiac function during fluid administration for hypovolemia, for infusion of caustic drugs and total parenteral nutrition (TPN), for air emboli aspiration, for insertion of pacing leads, and for venous access if peripheral veins are not adequate. Different approaches may be used (basilic, external jugular, subclavian, femoral), but the right internal jugular vein is commonly used because its use is associated with fewer complications. Catheters may be advanced over needles, through needles, or over a guidewire. The patient is usually sedated and is placed in the Trendelenburg position to distend the jugular vein and reduce the risks of air embolism. Local anesthetic (lidocaine) is used at the insertion site. Blood return indicates proper placement, which is confirmed by chest radiography. The catheter tip should not advance into the atrium. Complications include infection, thromboemboli, hematoma, pneumothorax, arrhythmias (if catheter is in right atrium), cardiac perforation or tamponade, and trauma. Most complications are related to poor technique.

## Cardioversion

**Cardioversion** is a timed electrical stimulation of the heart to convert a tachydysrhythmia (such as atrial fibrillation) to a normal sinus rhythm. Anticoagulation therapy is usually given for at least 3 weeks before elective cardioversion to reduce the risk of emboli, and digoxin is discontinued for at least 48 hours before the procedure. During the procedure, the patient is usually sedated, anesthetized (commonly with propofol, thiopental, methohexital, or etomidate), or both. Electrodes in the form of gel-covered paddles or pads are positioned on the left chest and the left back (in front of and behind the heart). These electrodes are connected by leads to a computerized ECG machine and a cardiac monitor with a defibrillator. The defibrillator is synchronized with the ECG so that the electrical current can be delivered during ventricular depolarization (QRS). The timing must be precise to prevent ventricular tachycardia or ventricular fibrillation. Drug therapy is sometimes used in conjunction with cardioversion; for example, antiarrhythmics (Cardizem, Cordarone) may be given before the procedure to slow the heart rate.

## Emergency defibrillation

**Emergency defibrillation** is performed to treat acute ventricular fibrillation or ventricular tachycardia in which there is no audible or palpable pulse. A higher voltage is generally used for defibrillation than for cardioversion, causing depolarization of myocardial cells, which can then repolarize to regain a normal sinus rhythm. Defibrillation delivers an electrical discharge, usually through paddles applied to both sides of the chest. Defibrillation may be repeated, usually as many as 3 times, at increasing voltage, but if the heart has not regained a sinus rhythm by then, cardiopulmonary resuscitation and advanced life support are required. Medications such as epinephrine or vasopressin may be administered, and cardiopulmonary resuscitation may be continued for one minute, after which defibrillation is again attempted. Additional medications, such as Cordarone, magnesium, or procainamide, may be necessary if ventricular dysrhythmias persist.

## Computed tomography (CT or CAT)

**Computed tomography (CT or CAT)** is a form of radiography that creates 2-dimensional (horizontal and vertical) cross-section images. Multiple x-ray beams and x-ray detectors rotate about the body, measuring the amount of absorbed radiation. The slices can be stacked to create a 3-dimensional image. A computer program translates the images into "slices," which can be displayed or printed. Oral, rectal, or intravenous contrast dye may be administered before the procedure because they cause blood vessels and hollow organs to appear brighter on images. This dye may cause a slight burning sensation in the arm, a metallic taste in the mouth, and a generalized feeling of warmth. These sensations subside within a few minutes. CT may be used for diagnosis, but it is often also used during surgical procedures to guide placement of catheters or needles, especially with minimally invasive procedures. CT requires less radiation than traditional radiography and provides more detail. It can be used to image any part of the body.

## Magnetic resonance imaging (MRI)

**Magnetic resonance imaging (MRI)** uses radio waves. A small body coil may be placed around the head or body part to send and receive the radio wave pulses. The energy from radio waves is absorbed and then released in a pattern formed by the type of tissue and by certain diseases. Intravenous contrast dye may be administered. Usually several sets of images are taken, each requiring 2 to 15 minute; therefore, a complete scan may take as long as an hour, although newer scanners are faster. MRI produces detailed images of organs and tissues from multiple planes. It provides images with greater contrast than CT; therefore, soft tissues are better visualized. MRI can evaluate hemorrhage, blood and CSF flow, tumors (differentiating them from normal tissue), edema, and damage to the structures inside a joint. Some surgical procedures, such as craniotomy, may be performed under MRI guidance. Children and the critically ill may require general anesthesia for MRI; an adult with claustrophobia may require sedation. An MRI-compatible fiberoptic pulse oximeter monitors oxygen saturation.

## Electroconvulsive therapy

**Electroconvulsive therapy** (ECT) is used primarily to treat depression but is also used to treat also bipolar disorder and other psychiatric diseases, usually when conventional medications, such as antidepressants, have been unsuccessful. The procedure requires approximately 20 minutes with therapeutic seizures lasting for approximately 30 to 60 seconds. Patients usually receive 2 to 3 treatments per week for a total of 3 to 12 treatments (400 to 700 seizure seconds). Electroconvulsive therapy may be applied to one side of the cerebrum, by placing two electrodes on the same side of the head, or to both sides of the cerebrum by placing the electrodes on opposite sides. Patients receive IV general anesthesia. Before induction, the patient receives 100% oxygen, and a BP cuff is placed around a distal limb (usually the lower leg or forearm) to prevent the muscle relaxants from affecting muscles distal to the cuff and to allow seizure activity to be monitored. A bite block is placed into the mouth. Induction is with methohexital, propofol, or etomidate alone or with esmolol, a rapid-acting opioid (remifentanil or alfentanil), or both.

Because most induction agents have antiseizure properties, small doses are given. To prevent musculoskeletal injury, succinylcholine or a short-acting nondepolarizing NMBA is given just before the electrical current is delivered. Supplemental oxygen is administered just before the treatment to prevent airway collapse, and the anesthetist displaces the mandible forward during the treatment. Seizure activity is monitored with EEG and by observing the unperfused extremity distal to the inflated cuff. The tonic phase (10 to 15 seconds) stimulates the parasympathetic system, causing bradycardia and sometimes hypotension. This is quickly followed by the clonic phase (30 to 60 seconds), which stimulates the sympathetic system and causes hypertension and tachycardia and sometimes arrhythmias, which abate after the convulsion ceases. Cerebral blood flow and ICP increase briefly. Hyperventilation may be used to increase the length of the seizure. Because treatment duration is short, the cardiovascular changes rarely require treatment. ECT is contraindicated for patients with intracranial lesions, those who have had a stroke within the past month, or those who have had a myocardial infarction within the past 3 months.

## Interventional radiology

**Interventional radiology** comprises neuroangiography and body angiography. Many minimally invasive procedures use angiographic guidance to determine areas of occlusion or abnormality and to place catheters and stents. Anticoagulation with heparin and antiplatelet agents (ASA, ticlopidine, glycoprotein antagonists) is often used to prevent thromboemboli. If heparinization is performed, then protamine (1 mg per 100 units of heparin activity) must be available to reverse anticoagulation in the event of hemorrhage. Local anesthesia with IV sedation is most commonly used, but general anesthesia may be used for some procedures. The patient must remain immobile, anticoagulation must be managed and monitored, and preparations must be made for complications, which can occur rapidly. Blood pressure must be maintained, sometimes at a hypertensive rate for thrombolysis and hemorrhage from subarachnoid aneurysm. Preventing hypertension may be crucial for those with recent rupture of an intracranial aneurysm, obliterated intracranial AV malformation, or existing stents in the carotid artery. Equipment for providing positive-pressure ventilation should be available during transit from the operating room.

## Electrophysiology

**Electrophysiology** is used for arrhythmias and heart block with a programmable pacemaker, an implanted cardioverter/defibrillator (ICD), or both. These procedures usually require local anesthesia and conscious sedation. Because it is important to avoid administering excessive IV fluids, a minidrip system may be used, and positive-pressure ventilation should be avoided so that increases in pulmonary vascular resistance can be prevented. Such increases decrease filling of the left ventricle and arterial pressure. Patients with a low ejection fraction may require monitoring with an arterial catheter. Low BP may be treated with phenylephrine or inotropes. Testing of timing parameters for the ICD includes repeated defibrillator tests, during which fibrillation is induced and then a shock is administered for defibrillation. During these procedures, it is important that the ECG monitor show pacemaker spikes; therefore, "show" must be set for pacemakers. Hand ventilation (gentle) with a mask may be used until spontaneous respiration recurs. For general anesthesia, induction is with etomidate supplemented with midazolam, and maintenance is with at least 50% nitrous oxide and a small amount of volatile anesthesia.

## Steroid therapy

**Steroid therapy** is given via an epidural to provide relief for back pain. It is most effective if given within 2 weeks of the onset of pain related to neural compression and inflammation. Steroids (methylprednisolone 40-80 mg or triamcinolone diacetate 40-80mg) are given with saline or a local anesthetic, which provides pain relief until the steroid takes effect in 12 to 48 hours. However, epidural local anesthetics pose a higher risk of complications related to intrathecal, intravascular, or subdural administration. This problem may be obviated by using fluoroscopic guidance for insertion of the needle and confirming placement with epidurography. A transforaminal epidural approach is more effective than a translaminar approach. As with other epidurals, a caudal injection may be necessary for those who have had back surgery. The needle should be cleared of steroid before withdrawal to prevent development of fistula. Spinal administration is contraindicated because the preservative ethylene glycol may cause adhesions.

## Radiation therapy

**Radiation therapy** includes treatments with instruments such as the CyberKnife and the Gamma Knife. CyberKnife treatments may require no anesthesia or may require mild conscious sedation, depending on the patient. The anesthetist must be sure to keep the anesthesia equipment away from the robotic arms of the machine. The patient is positioned according to the area being irradiated. The Gamma Knife is used only on the head to treat intracranial tumors and AVMs; it is more uncomfortable than the CyberKnife because it requires a stereotactic frame. Patients are given local anesthetic at the sites in the skull at which the stereotactic frame is attached. Patients younger than 12 years usually receive general anesthesia; older patients receive IV sedation (midazolam and fentanyl) as needed. After the frame has been attached, the patient undergoes angiography and MRI or CT (or both) and is then taken to a recovery area to await results before the procedure. During radiation delivery for both treatments, medical staff are in a shielded control area, and the patient is monitored with videos.

## Endoscopy

**Endoscopy** comprises laryngoscopy, microlaryngoscopy (with microscope), esophagoscopy, and bronchoscopy. If there is upper airway obstruction, the patient should not receive premedication sedatives. Glycopyrrolate may be given 1 hour preoperatively to reduce secretions. Muscle relaxation with continuous succinylcholine or intermittent administration of short-acting nondepolarizing NMBAs keeps the area immobile. Ventilation is usually achieved with a small tracheal tube (4.0-6.0 mm) and positive pressure, but because these tubes are too short for adults, a

4.0- to 6.0-mm microlaryngeal tracheal tube (MLT) may be used. Intubation protects against aspiration and allows monitoring of end-tidal $CO_2$. Another approach alternates 2- to 3-minute periods of apnea (when surgery is performed) with periods of ventilation, but this procedure risks hypoventilation, hypercarbia, and pulmonary aspiration. A manual jet ventilator may be connected to a side port to provide high-pressure oxygen during inspiration. Heart rate and BP may fluctuate during the procedures; therefore, supplemental administration of short-acting anesthetics and esmolol may maintain stability. A regional nerve block (glossopharyngeal and superior laryngeal) also minimizes blood pressure variations.

## Management of anesthetic and surgical complications

### Anesthesia-related

**Complications** related to anesthesia and surgery:

- Malfunction of breathing circuits, monitors, ventilator, anesthesia machine, and laryngoscope.
- Accidental disconnection of breathing circuit; inappropriate use of anesthesia machine. Drug/fluid volume errors.
- Incorrect placement of IV or epidurals.
- Airway injury: Dental trauma is most common, but laryngeal injuries can include paralysis of vocal cords, granuloma, and arytenoid dislocation. Tracheal injuries usually relate to tracheotomies rather than intubation. Esophageal and pharyngoesophageal perforation can occur, often associated with a late onset of symptoms.
- Peripheral nerve trauma, such as ulnar neuropathy, can occur with general and regional anesthesia. Injury may also relate to incorrect positioning or cushioning of the body.
- Hypotension and air embolism.
- Compartment syndrome may result from venous obstruction or vascular puncture with hemorrhage.
- Eye injury may result from corneal abrasion or ischemic optic neuropathy, and low-frequency hearing loss may result after dural puncture and CSF leaks. Awareness during anesthesia.
- Cardiac arrest related to spinal anesthesia and α-agonist/β-blocker interaction.

## Trauma management issues

Trauma victims may arrive in the operating room with a number of unique **management issues**:

- *Gastric emptying* is delayed after trauma, and all victims are treated as though they have a full stomach. If an NG tube is in place, it should be set to suction, but this does not preclude aspiration. Rapid-sequence induction should be performed with cricoid pressure.
- *Cervical injury* may result in further injury or paralysis if spinal precautions are not used. A Bullard laryngoscope should be used, or, if the patient is awake, fiberoptic intubation may be used.
- *Substance abuse* (drugs or alcohol) is common among trauma patients (≤50%). Such abuse can affect anesthesia management, depending on the type of substance and the amount of ingestion; anesthetic requirements may be altered, and blood pressure and recovery may be affected.
- *Fluid loss*, especially from bleeding, may contribute to hypovolemia, because vasoconstriction increases the concentration of drugs.

- *Slowing metabolism* affects clearance of drugs through liver and kidneys, prolonging action of anesthetics.
- *Pelvic fractures* are associated with a high mortality rate and require ongoing fluid resuscitation.

## Anesthesia

Many issues are related to **anesthesia with trauma**:

- Induction: If hypotension related to hypovolemia is present, then volume replacement should be performed before induction if possible. Thiopental and propofol should be avoided. Opioids may increase hypotension. Ketamine and etomidate are often drugs of choice. Ketamine can be used with hypovolemia but can cause increased intracranial pressure (ICP); therefore, it must be avoided for patients with head injury. Etomidate may be used for patients with hypotension.
- Because low doses of anesthetic agent are often used, patients often require NMDA; however, there drugs increase awareness during surgery. Scopolamine 5 to 10 mcg/kg or intermittent doses of midazolam may be used as an amnesic agent.
- Nitrous oxide is usually avoided with trauma. It should not be used for patients with pneumothorax, closed head injuries, bowel injury, or air emboli.
- Positive-pressure ventilation may cause a tension pneumothorax (tachycardia, hypotension, jugular vein distention, and absence of breath sounds on the affected side) and may necessitate placement of a large-bore needle for decompression until a chest tube can be inserted.

## Hemorrhage

**Hemorrhage** associated with trauma often involves the loss of 30% or more of blood volume, resulting in hypovolemic shock, organ hypoperfusion, and ischemic necrosis. At 30% loss, symptoms become obvious: restlessness, confusion, thirst, and pallor. This begins the nonprogressive stage of hypovolemic shock. Initially, in the nonprogressive stage, the body compensates with sympathetic stimulation (tachycardia, vasoconstriction, renal conservation), but as the progressive stage takes over, tissue hypoxia causes increased lactic acidosis and decreased tissue pH. Disseminated intravascular coagulation (DIC) can occur, and kidneys begin to shut down. In the last stage, extensive injury to tissue results in myocardial depression and renal failure with acute tubular necrosis. To prevent this deterioration, fluid resuscitation must be immediate and aggressive. Crystalloids are usually given initially, but with severe hemorrhage (30%-40%) blood products must be administered. All fluids and blood products are warmed to prevent hypothermia. Protocols for massive blood replacement should be followed, including giving one unit of plasma with each unit of PRBCs to help prevent coagulopathy.

## Cardiac tamponade

**Cardiac tamponade** is heart compression due to collection of blood in the pericardium; it prevents filling, especially of the thin-walled atria. Cardiac tamponade may be indicated by Beck's triad: jugular venous distention, hypotension, and muffled heart tones upon auscultation (including friction rub). Hypotension, tachycardia, and tachypnea usually occur rapidly. Pulsus paradoxus is usually evident. Heart size may appear normal on radiography; ECG indications may be nonspecific ST-segment and T-wave abnormalities. Two-dimensional echocardiography is effective in allowing estimates of the size of effusion. The effusion must be evacuated surgically or with pericardiocentesis (which poses risks of pneumothorax and cardiac or coronary artery laceration). Anesthesia depends on the circumstances, but ketamine is usually used for induction, and succinylcholine or pancuronium is used for maintenance. There is an increased risk for cardiac collapse on induction, therefore pericardiocentesis is with local anesthetic and should be performed before induction if possible, but general anesthesia and intubation are used for surgical approaches. Intravenous access must be available for fluid replacement. Anesthesia should avoid vasodilation, bradycardia, or cardiac depression. Thoracoscopy requires one-lung anesthesia.

## Burn injuries

### General management

**General management of burn injuries** must include both wound care and systemic care to avoid complications that can be life threatening. Treatment includes establishment of airway and treatment for inhalation injury as indicated, supplemental oxygen, incentive spirometry, nasotracheal suctioning, humidification, bronchoscopy as needed to evaluate bronchospasm and edema, β-agonists for bronchospasm followed by aminophylline if ineffective, and intubation and ventilation if there are indications of respiratory failure. This should be performed before failure. Tracheostomy may be performed if ventilation is required for more than 14 days. Focus on fluid resuscitation, due to increase in capillary permeability leading to fluid shifting to interstitial space so give intravenous fluids and electrolytes, administered in amounts based on weight and extent of burn. Parkland formula: 4 mL per kg body weight × %BSA for the first 24 hours. Enteral feedings, usually with small-lumen feeding tube into the duodenum. NG tube for gastric decompression to prevent aspiration. Indwelling catheter to monitor urinary output. Urinary output should be 0.5 to 2 mL/kg/hr. Analgesia for reduction of pain and anxiety. Topical and systemic antibiotics. Wound care with removal of eschar and dressings as indicated.

### Anesthetic management

**Anesthetic management of burn injuries** depends on the type and extent of burns:

- General anesthesia is used for escharotomy, excision, and grafting. Standard procedures are used if there is no damage to airways, but patients with inhalational injuries may already be intubated before surgery because of hypoxia and upper-airway edema or secretions. Fiberoptic intubation of awake patients may be necessary with contractures or impending airway obstruction.
- Continuous monitoring of pulmonary function is crucial because function may be severely compromised by direct inhalational injury or secondary pulmonary response. Compliance may decrease with burns about the thorax.
- Volatile anesthetics may initially increase cardiac depression but may be used after the acute phase.
- Dressings soaked in epinephrine may be used to decrease blood loss.
- 100% oxygen or hyperbaric oxygen may be needed for patients who have inhaled carbon monoxide or hydrogen cyanide. Additionally, hypermetabolism associated with burns increases oxygen consumption.
- Succinylcholine is contraindicated after the first 24 hours because it may cause cardiac arrest and hyperkalemia. It should be recognized that there is often resistance to NDMR in this population, causing the patient to need up to five times the normal dose.
- Skin excision often causes extensive blood loss, especially if treatment is delayed for a few days or if burns are extensive; therefore, fluids must be replaced as needed, using the Parkland formula as appropriate.
- Urinary output should be measured with a Foley catheter to ensure output of 1 mL/kg/hr. Dopamine may be used.
- Heat loss is common and should be monitored carefully and controlled with heated blankets or heat lamps, increased ambient temperature, and warmed IV fluids.

- Monitoring should include ECG with needle electrodes as necessary, pulmonary artery catheter, and central venous catheter. Triple-lumen catheters may be used for difficult intravenous access because of damaged tissue.
- Electrolytes should be monitored because some topical medications, such as silver nitrate, may alter electrolyte balance.
- Electrical burns cause myoglobinuria that can cause renal failure.

## Cardiopulmonary resuscitation

### Cardiac arrest with ventricular fibrillation or tachycardia

**Cardiopulmonary resuscitation** has the same basic underlying treatments, but there are at times specific interventions based on patient indications (i.e., giving rapid incrementally increasing doses of epi to a patient in arrest during subarachnoid block). Cardiac arrest is the complete absence of pulse and may be caused by ventricular fibrillation, ventricular tachycardia, pulseless electrical activity (PEA), and asystole. The immediate response, regardless of cause, is to begin CPR, provide oxygen, and attach a defibrillator. Treatment for ***ventricular fibrillation*** or ***ventricular tachycardia*** includes the following:

1. A shock is delivered and CPR is resumed.
2. If the condition persists, another shock is administered and epinephrine 1 mg (repeated every 3-5 minutes) is administered; vasopressin 40 U may be substituted for the first or second dose. This continues for as many as 5 CPR cycles. Note: One cycle of CPR comprises 30 compressions and 2 breaths.
3. At this point, another shock is administered, CPR is resumed, and antiarrhythmics, such as amiodarone 300 mg and then 150 mg or lidocaine 1 to 1.5 mg/kg and then 0.5 to 0.75 mg/kg (to 3 doses), are administered. Magnesium (1-2 g) may be administered. This continues for 5 CPR cycles. The cycle is then repeated from step 2 until normal heart rhythm resumes or a decision is made to discontinue resuscitation.

### Cardiac arrest with asystole

**Cardiac arrest with asystole** is treated with cardiopulmonary resuscitation. Note: One cycle of CPR comprises 30 compressions and 2 breaths. Five cycles require approximately 2 minutes, after which rhythm checks are performed. If an advanced airway is in place, 8 to 10 breaths per minute are given with continuous chest compressions. Cardiac arrest related to ***pulseless electrical activity (PEA), asystole***, unlike that related to ventricular fibrillation or tachycardia, does not respond to shock. CPR with supplementary oxygen (if available) is begun immediately, and the following cycle of treatment is begun:

1. CPR for 5 cycles and then epinephrine 1 mg every 3 to 5 minutes; the first or second dose of epinephrine may be replaced with vasopressin 40 U. Atropine 1 mg may be given every 3 to 5 minutes (≤3 doses).
2. If asystole continues, step 1 is repeated.
3. If shockable rhythm begins, a shock is given and CPR is resumed. At this point, the procedure follows that for ventricular fibrillation or ventricular tachycardia.
4. If normal (non-shockable) rhythm begins, postresuscitation care is begun.

## Symptomatic bradycardia

Cardiopulmonary resuscitation is performed to treat **symptomatic bradycardia**, a heart rate lower than 60 bpm that causes serious adverse symptoms. The patient is given supplementary oxygen, and the airway is checked to ensure patency. ECG, BP, and oxygen saturation are monitored, and IV access must be established if not already available. The patient is evaluated for evidence of decreased perfusion:

- If perfusion appears to be adequate, then the patient is monitored.
- If there are indications of poor perfusion (hypotension, shock, chest pain, changes in mentation), then the patient should be prepared for transcutaneous pacing. Atropine 0.5 mg, epinephrine 2 to 20 µg/min, or dopamine 1-20 µg/kg per minute may be given before the pacer is available.

The patient should be evaluated for conditions that may contribute to bradycardia, such as hypovolemia, hypoxia, toxins, tension pneumothorax, hypothermia, thrombosis, metabolic acidosis, hypoglycemia, or hypokalemia.

Symptomatic tachycardia

**Symptomatic tachycardia** must be evaluated with ECG to determine whether the QRS segment is narrow or wide, because this affects the treatment protocol. Once tachycardia has been detected, oxygen is provided and an effort is made to identify and reverse the causes. If the patient's condition appears stable, an IV must be established and a 12-lead ECG obtained. If the patient's condition is unstable, IV access and sedation are given and immediate cardioversion is performed, even if the patient remains conscious:

- *Narrow QRS with regular rhythm* is treated with vagal maneuvers and adenosine 6 mg IV push, followed by 12 mg ×X 2 if no conversion. If conversion takes place, the patient must be carefully monitored and treated again for recurrence. If the rhythm does not convert, β-blockers may be used (with caution if CHF or pulmonary disease is present).
- *Narrow QRS with irregular rhythm* (atrial fibrillation, flutter, or multifocal atrial tachycardia) is treated with β-blockers.
- *Wide QRS with regular rhythm* (ventricular tachycardia or uncertain rhythm) is treated with amiodarone 150 mg IV over 10 minutes, repeated to a maximum dose of 2.2 g for 24 hours, and elective synchronized cardioversion. If supraventricular tachycardia occurs, this is treated as for narrow QRS.
- *Wide QRS with irregular rhythm* is treated according to the types of irregularity. If atrial fibrillation with aberrancy, it is treated as for irregular narrow QRS tachycardia. If preexcited atrial fibrillation, antiarrhythmics, such as amiodarone 250 mg IV, may be given over 10 minutes. AV blocking agents should be avoided. Recurrent polymorphic ventricular tachycardia requires cardiac consultation. *Torsades de pointes* are treated with magnesium 1-2 g over 5-60 minutes and then infusion.

Contributing factors should be determined. These include hypovolemia, hypoxia, metabolic acidosis, hypoglycemia, hypokalemia, hyperkalemia, hypothermia, toxins, cardiac tamponade, tension pneumothorax, and thrombosis.

**Pacemaker insertion**

**Pacemakers** are inserted with a minimally invasive technique that requires a subclavicular incision approximately 3 inches long in the left upper chest to create a pocket for the pacemaker in the tissue over the muscle. Endocardial leads are threaded through a major vein into the right ventricle, and epicardial leads (always temporary) are sutured to the outside of the heart and brought through the chest wall during open heart surgery. Endocardial leads are most commonly inserted through the external jugular vein and are connected to the generator implanted in the chest wall. This procedure is usually performed in a cardiac catheterization laboratory and requires local anesthesia and sometimes mild sedation. The procedure usually lasts approximately 45 minutes. After surgery, the pacemaker is programmed with an external programming device. Cardiac function is monitored with ECG, and a defibrillator must be available to administer shock or transcutaneous pacing if sudden arrest or bradycardia occurs. In general placing a magnet over a pacemaker stops the pacemaker from sensing and causes asynchronous pacing at a preprogrammed rate.

## Lithotripsy

**Lithotripsy**, the use of shock waves to pulverize kidney stones, is commonly used instead of open surgical removal of kidney stones. Patients with a pacemaker, an implanted cardiac defibrillator, or a history of arrhythmias may develop shock-induced arrhythmias; therefore, the manufacturer's instructions should be followed regarding reprogramming the device or applying a magnet. To prevent arrhythmias, the shocks may be synchronized with the R wave of an ECG so that the shock occurs 20 ms after the R wave (ventricular refractory period). Because hematuria is common as a result of the shock, monitoring for bleeding, hematoma, and thrombus formation is necessary.

A number of different procedures are used:

- *Cystoscopic procedures* with ureteroscopy, extraction of stone, placement of stents, and intracorporeal lithotripsy laser (holmium:YAG laser) are commonly performed for bladder or ureteral stones. Anesthetic management is similar to that for other cystoscopic procedures.
- *Extracorporeal shock wave lithotripsy* (ESWL) uses short-duration shock waves to pulverize calculi. Shock waves are generated from water-filled cushions on a special table. A conducting gel on the skin transmits the shock waves. With this type of lithotripsy, pain is usually mild and is managed with short-acting drugs. Ureteral stents may be placed with cystoscopy before this procedure. IV sedation with midazolam and opioids are usually sufficient for anesthesia.
- *Immersion lithotripsy* places the patient in a hydraulic chair, which is then immersed in heated water, and shock waves are generated electromagnetically or with piezoelectric crystals. This procedure can cause vasodilation and hypotension and is extremely painful; therefore, patients require regional (continuous epidural) or general anesthesia with intubation (which poses management problems) or light general anesthesia with NMBAs. To prevent hypotension, IV loading with 1000 mL of lactated Ringer's is used before patients are placed upright in a chair.

### Organ transplantation

<u>Heart</u>

**Heart transplantation** requires cardiopulmonary bypass (CPB) with anesthetic considerations similar to those for other open heart procedures. Due to the negative inotropic effect of anesthesia, heart transplant patients are at an increased risk for CV collapse, and their anesthesia requires diligent and judicious selection and titration of agents. Ventricular assist devices prior to transplantation are becoming more common as well. After sternotomy, the pericardial sac is opened to expose the heart. If the donor heart is larger than the recipient's, the left pericardium may be removed, sparing the phrenic nerve. The *orthotopic* procedure is most common: The posterior portion of the left and right atrium (with caval and pulmonary vein openings) is left for attachment of the new heart. The donor heart may be trimmed and is sutured to fit the remnants of the old heart. Once the donor heart has been sutured, ventricle function, rhythm, and coagulation status is monitored and corrected as needed. Once stable, CPB is discontinued, and the heart is

- 79 -

stimulated to begin contractions. Methylprednisolone is administered before the aortic cross-clamp is removed. Isoproterenol is usually given before CPB is discontinued. If right ventricular failure occurs because of pulmonary hypertension, hyperventilation, prostaglandin, and nitric oxide may be administered, and a right ventricular assist device (RVAD) may be used, as the right ventricle's function is key in being able to come off pump after transplant.

Lung

**Lung transplantation** is the replacement of one or both lungs, and sometimes a lobe, with donor organs. Combined heart and lung transplants are much less common now than previously. Lung transplantation is often indicated because of end-stage parenchymal damage to the lungs caused by COPD, cystic fibrosis, pulmonary fibrosis, or pulmonary hypertension. Single-lung transplantation is usually performed for COPD, but double-lung transplantation is used for cystic fibrosis, bullous emphysema, or vascular diseases of the lungs. Premedication includes oral cyclosporine, but sedation is usually withheld until the patient is in the operating room. Azathioprine may be given before induction. Invasive monitoring is similar to that used for cardiac surgery. Induction is performed with the patient in the supine position, with the head slightly elevated. Ketamine, etomidate, or opioid (or combination) may be used for slow induction. Succinylcholine or a nondepolarizing NMBA may be used to facilitate laryngoscopy, with constant cricoid pressure. Hypoxemia and hypercapnia can cause increased pulmonary artery pressure; therefore, patients must be monitored and treated.

Hypotension is treated with dobutamine rather than IV bolus. Maintenance is by IV opioid infusion, sometimes with a low-dose inhalational volatile agent. Procedures include the following:

- **Single-lung transplantation:** This procedure uses a posterior thoracotomy and may be performed with or without CPB, depending on patient response. If there is persistent arterial hypoxemia ($Spo_2$ <88%) or increased pulmonary artery pressure, then CPB is initiated with femoral-vein-to-femoral-artery bypass during right thoracotomy. The recipient lung is removed, and the donor lung is anastomosed.
- **Double-lung transplantation:** This procedure uses a transverse sternotomy and either normothermic CPB or sequential thoracotomy without CPB (more common). IV hydrochloric acid may be needed to treat severe metabolic alkalosis in patients with marked $CO_2$ retention.

When the donor lung or lungs are anastomosed, ventilation is resumed with an inspired oxygen concentration of less than 60%. Methylprednisolone is given before vascular clamps are released. If the results of coagulation studies are normal, a thoracic epidural catheter may be used for pain control postoperatively.

**Heart or heart-lung transplantation risk factors**

Patients undergoing **heart or heart-lung transplant** are especially susceptible to bacterial pulmonary infections, which occur in 35% to 48% of hosts. Some factors place patients at increased risk:

- **CMV-positive donor** places seronegative patients undergoing heart, lung, or heart-lung transplant at increased risk of postoperative CMV pneumonia, invasive aspergillosis, and pulmonary bacterial infections.
- **Preoperative colonization of Aspergillus fumigatus** in cystic fibrosis patients poses the risk of postoperative tracheobronchial aspergillosis.

- 80 -

- **Colonization of resistant Pseudomonas strains** in the damaged lungs, especially in cystic fibrosis patients, can result in residual infection in other parts of the respiratory tract, providing a source of infection for the donor organs.
- **Invasive devices** such as central venous lines, circulatory assist devices, and ventilators may result in colonization and infection, especially pneumonia and sternal surgical site infections.
- **Decreased ability to cough and clear mucous** because of loss of cough reflex, pain, or weakness can contribute to the incidence of pneumonia.

## Liver transplantation

**Liver transplantation** is often the only effective treatment for end-stage liver disease or abnormalities (extrahepatic biliary atresia), metabolic diseases (Wilson's disease), toxic necrosis (viral infections, drugs), cirrhosis, and malignancies. There are three stages of liver transplantation: preanhepatic, anhepatic, and reperfusion. During the preanhepatic stage, focus is on warming the patient, correcting electrolyte levels, treating hypovolemia secondary to blood loss, and correcting coagulapathies. During the anhepatic stage there is continual concern with monitoring electrolytes and monitoring volume status. During the postanhepatic stage bleeding, coagulopathies, labile pressures, and arrhythmias are anticipated and corrected. At this point graft function can be assessed. On presentation for surgery patients may appear hyperdynamic hemodynamically, with an increased CI and decreased SVR, however many times they have cardiac dysfunction, CAD, and pulmonary hypertension. Anesthetic management includes monitoring of arterial blood pressure and central venous pressure (CVP) and may include transesophageal echocardiography (TEE). Nitrous oxide is avoided, although a number of drugs can be used for induction and maintenance even though some may be excreted through the liver.

## Kidney transplantation

**Kidney transplantation** is indicated for a wide range of disorders, including kidney disease requiring dialysis, congenital abnormalities with urinary blockage, glomerulonephritis, and hemolytic uremic syndrome. Diabetes is the primary cause of kidney disease requiring transplantation. Adult cadaveric or living donor organs (47%) may be used. Usually the diseased kidney is not removed; therefore, the donor kidney is placed in a different position, usually in the iliac fossa. Steroids, such as prednisone, have been used with tacrolimus for immunosuppression, but the results of recent studies indicate that the extended use of daclizumab can provide equally effective steroid-free immunosuppression, with fewer adverse effects. Other studies have shown that preconditioning with alemtuzumab and tacrolimus allows avoidance of steroids. Anesthetic management is as for renal failure and may include preoperative dialysis. General anesthesia is used with extensive monitoring (especially in diabetic patients) to maintain CVP between 10 and 15 mm Hg. Opioids are used sparingly to prevent hypotension, and $\alpha$-adrenergic drugs are avoided because they may contribute to compromised blood flow in the transplanted kidney.

## Pancreas transplantation

**Pancreas transplantation** is performed to treat type 1 insulin-dependent diabetes mellitus. Because of the danger of rejection and the need for immunosuppressive drugs, transplantation is usually reserved for patients with severe symptoms. Pancreas grafts are obtained from cadaveric or living donors who have undergone surgical removal of half of the pancreas. Most pancreas transplants (85%) are performed in conjunction with kidney transplants or after kidney transplants (10%) because of kidney damage caused by diabetes. Many patients are receiving dialysis before surgery. Another procedure that is still fairly new is islet transplantation, which involves isolating islet cells from a donor organ and then transplanting them by infusion into the portal vein of the liver. Patients often require 2 or 3 transplants, but some achieve insulin independence. This procedure is still considered experimental but shows promise. Both pancreas and islet cell transplantations require immunosuppression.

## Living donor (renal) organ procurement

Procurement of a **kidney** from a **living donor** requires general anesthesia with intubation for open surgery or laparoscopy; the patient is placed in the lateral decubitus position. Induction is usually performed with propofol (2-3 mg/kg), but thiopental or etomidate may also be used. A nondepolarizing NMBA (vecuronium) and an opioid (fentanyl) are also used. If the donor has acid reflux, rapid-sequence induction is used along with succinylcholine. Maintenance is usually with balanced anesthesia (isoflurane or desflurane with 50% $O_2$ and fentanyl). Sevoflurane and nitrous oxide are usually avoided for donors. Mannitol is administered to the donor. In some cases, spinal-epidural anesthesia is used. The kidney must be monitored to limit ischemia; therefore, perfusion must be sufficient during procurement, and heparins should be administered immediately before harvesting to avoid thrombosis. The anesthetist helps to prepare the kidney by providing adequate oxygen and hydration during dissection. Upon induction, 10 mL/kg Ringer's lactate should be administered; additional boluses may be administered as needed to maintain urinary output and BP stability until the kidney has been harvested.

## Living donor (liver) organ procurement

Procurement of part of the **liver** from a **living donor** requires a right hepatic lobectomy (adequate for adult recipient), which includes removal of the gallbladder, or a left hepatic lobectomy, a less complicated procedure (adequate for pediatric recipients). Anesthesia is similar to that for kidney procurement with the donor in the lateral decubitus position, but because liver procurement may involve significant blood loss (0.5-1 L), large-bore IV access must be available for fluid replacement and, in some cases, transfusions. (Donors are often asked to bank 2 units of blood before the transplant.) Low central venous pressure anesthesia (<5 mm Hg) is used to decrease cardiac filling pressures. After the resection, a typical reaction is a decrease in vascular resistance with an increase in heart rate and cardiac output. In some cases epidural catheters are placed for postoperative pain control, but this may pose a slight problem because temporary coagulopathies may occur postoperatively; therefore, clotting times are monitored carefully. Complications include metabolic acidosis, respiratory impairment, and pneumothorax.

## Cadaver procurement

Cadaveric procurement of organs is done with **non-heart-beating cadavers** or **heart-beating cadavers**:

- *Non-heart-beating donors* are typically those who have died circulatory deaths and are maintained on life support until transported to the operating room where life support is discontinued, interrupting blood supply to the organs, which are then harvested. Ethical issues have arisen about anesthetists being present, suggesting that the person is still alive and needs anesthetic care. Thus, anesthetists are usually not involved in this type of procurement.

- However, with ***heart-beating cadavers***, the donor is brain dead but is maintained on life support until procurement of organs in complete. The anesthetist must manage all body systems to ensure that organs are perfused. This may require administration of intravenous fluids, packed red blood cells, and vasopressor or inotropic agents to manage blood pressure, although overload must be avoided. High-dose steroids may be used, for example to improve lung donor recovery. Inspired O2 concentration is usually less than 50% and positive end-expiratory pressure (PEEP) is less than 5 cm $H_2O$, especially if lungs are to be donated.

## Lasers use

**Laser** use is often combined with endoscopy. Laser use is determined by wavelength, which corresponds to the medium in which it is generated. $CO_2$ lasers have a long wavelength, whereas YAG (yttrium-aluminum-garnet) lasers have a shorter wavelength. The shorter the wavelength, the deeper the tissue penetration. Many lasers require protective eye gear for medical staff and for the patient, whose eyes are taped shut. Intermittent ventilation or jet ventilation is often used to avoid tracheal tube fire. Additionally, a laser-resistant tracheal tube should be used, such as a flexible stainless steel tube. (Wrapping tubes in metallic tape is not safe.) Since no cuffed tracheal tube is completely safe, the following precautions must be used:

- Maintain inspired oxygen concentration as low as possible (many tolerate Fio2 of 21%).
- Use air or helium in place of nitrous oxide.
- Fill tracheal tube cuffs with saline dyed with methylene blue to dissipate heat and signal rupture.
- Place saline-soaked pledgets in the airway.
- Keep 60 mL syringe of water available.

# Pediatrics

## Pediatric anatomy, physiology, and pathophysiology

### Respiratory system
**Infants and children** have a number of anatomic and physiological differences that must be accounted for during administration of anesthesia. These differences are especially related to the **respiratory system**. Neonates and infants have relatively few small airways and alveoli; thus, airway resistance is increased and lung compliance is decreased. The rib cage (which is cartilaginous) is more compliant, causing collapse of the chest wall during inspiration and low residual expiratory volumes with decreased functional residual capacity. Maturation of alveoli does not occur until the age of approximately 8 years. Chest wall muscles are underdeveloped and weak. Additionally, a child's metabolic consumption of oxygen is twice that of an adult. The respiratory rate in a neonate is about 40/min; at the age of one year it is 30/min. It does not reach the normal adult rate of 20/min until the child reaches the age of 12. Furthermore, hypoxia and hypercapnia depress respirations in neonates and infants. This makes the child more prone to hypoxemia.

Airway

A number of important factors are related to the **pediatric airway**:

- Anatomic differences in infants make them obligate nasal breathers until about 5 months of age.
- The infant's head and tongue are proportionately large, the neck short, and the nasal passages narrow, resulting in a larynx that is anterior and cephalad, an elongated epiglottis, and a short trachea. The narrow airway increases the danger of obstruction, and even minimal edema can be obstructive.
- The larynx is adjacent to C4 and does not assume the adult position (adjacent to C6) until the child reaches the age of 6. The narrowest point in the airway of children under 5 years old is the cricoid cartilage (in older children and adults it is the glottis).
- The branching of the right main bronchus is at a 55° angle; in adults, it is at a 25° angle. Additionally, adenoids and tonsils are often quite prominent.

Because of the narrow airway, infants and children are more prone to laryngospasm and postintubation croup (especially those aged 1-4 years). Other factors that can contribute to postintubation croup include difficult intubation requiring multiple attempts, incorrect ETT size (too large), instability of ETT with excessive movement, and prolonged surgery. Postintubation croup is treated with nebulized racemic epinephrine in normal saline. The difficult airway makes choosing an age-appropriate ETT very important. The following formula is used to estimate ETT sizes: (age in years + 16) ÷ 4 = ETT size (internal diameter in mm). Usually, the depth to which an ETT can be inserted is estimated at 3 times the internal diameter of the ETT (or 12 + age ÷ 2 = length). An acceptable ETT leak is 15 to 20 cm $H_2O$ pressure. If a leak occurs at higher pressure, a smaller ETT should be used to avoid trauma and airway edema.

Cardiovascular system

There are a number of **pediatric cardiovascular** considerations. Because the left ventricle in neonates and infants is relatively noncompliant, stroke volume does not vary; thus, cardiac output directly relates to the heart rate. The infant's heart rate is faster than the adult's, and arterial blood pressure is lower. The approximate normal values follow (may vary):

0 = HR, 140 bpm; BP, 65/40 mm Hg
1 yr = HR, 125 bpm; BP, 95/60 mm Hg
3 yrs = HR, 100 bpm; BP, 100/70 mm Hg
9 yrs = HR, 80 bpm; BP, 105/70 mm Hg
12 yrs = HR, 80 bpm; BP, 110/60 mm Hg

The sympathetic nervous system is not well developed, and the parasympathetic system may be activated, resulting in bradycardia, also contributed to by excess anesthesia and hypoxia. The result is that infants and small children are prone to decreased cardiac output, hypotension, and asystole. The heart is more responsive to calcium channel blocking properties of volatile anesthetics. The vascular system does not respond to hypovolemia with adequate vasoconstriction, so indications of fluid depletion include hypotension without tachycardia.

The foramen ovale is an opening between the right and left atria. During fetal development, this opening allows blood to flow from the right atrium to the left atrium. The ductus arteriosus connects the pulmonary artery to the aortic arch so that fetal blood from the right atrium bypasses the lungs. The foramen ovale and ductus arteriosus open during fetal circulation and for as long as 4 months after birth, may have increased shunting of blood in the presence of hypoxemia and acidosis in infants younger than 4 months because these conditions cause an increase in pulmonary vascular resistance, resulting in increased right-to-left shunt and increasing hypoxemia. This creates a spiraling cycle of increased shunting. Additionally, reductions in systemic vascular resistance and hypothermia (from production of norepinephrine or non-shivering thermogenesis) may cause increased right-to-left shunting through the foramen ovale and ductus arteriosus because of pulmonary vasoconstriction.

Thermoregulation

A number of anatomic and physiological factors affect **pediatric thermoregulation.** Infants and children have larger body surface/weight ratios than adults, thinner skin, and lower fat content. Infants can produce heat only by activity, shivering (if older than 3 months), and nonshivering thermogenesis. Approximately 5% of infants' weight is composed of brown fat, so called because is highly vascularized and contains unmyelinated neurons that respond to sympathetic stimulation. The amount of brown fat decreases with age and is not present in adults. The lipid reserves in brown fat deplete in the presence of cold, causing the brown fat to darken. When an infant is exposed to cold, brown adipocytes (the cells of brown fat) respond to sympathetic stimulation and production of norepinephrine by oxidizing fatty acids and producing heat in a process called non-shivering thermogenesis. However, brown fat metabolism is impaired in infants who are premature or underweight, with inadequate stores of fat. Additionally, this thermogenesis is inhibited by volatile anesthetics.

Other factors that contribute to hypothermia in infants and small children are decreased temperature in the operating wound, exposure of the wound to ambient temperature, and intravenous fluid administration. The anesthetist must ensure that measures are taken to prevent hypothermia. These measures can include the following:

- Maintaining ambient temperature of 26°C.
- Using warming mattresses. These are useful only for small infants because older children do not have enough body contact with the mattress to effect warming. Fluid or air-heated blankets may be used for older children.
- Using forced-air (convective) warmers.
- Applying a plastic head covering to reduce heat loss through evaporation.

Induced hypothermia may be used for some procedures, such as open-heart procedures with cardiopulmonary bypass (CPB), but core temperatures must be carefully monitored.

Renal system and fluid maintenance

The pediatric **renal system** matures over the first 3 years of life. The nephrons in the young infant's kidneys are immature, and the glomerular filtration rate is low because of impaired ability to filter urine until the infant reaches 6 to 12 months of age. Also, the ability to concentrate or dilute urine may not reach adult levels until the child is 2 to 3 years old. Premature infants may have additional renal abnormalities, such as decreased creatinine clearance or impaired sodium retention. Infants are less tolerant of both dehydration and fluid overload. These factors make *maintenance of adequate fluid volume* more difficult during surgical procedures. The 4-2-1 rule is used to determine maintenance fluid requirements:

- 4 mL/kg/hr for the first 10 kg weight, 2 mL/kg/hr for the second 10 kg, and 1 mL/kg/hr for remaining weight.

Often a programmable infusion pump or buret with microdrip is used to manage fluids because the balance must be maintained within a narrow range.

Fluid deficit

**Pediatric fluid deficit** must also be carefully estimated and managed. Fluid deficit should be replaced over a period of 3 hours with half given during the first hour and a quarter given during each of the remaining 2 hours. Fluid deficit is calculated by first finding the ***maintenance fluid requirement***:

- Maintenance fluid mL × hours NPO = fluid deficit.

Preoperative deficits are usually treated with lactated Ringer's or 1/ normal saline (which may cause hyperchloremic acidosis). Glucose-containing fluids may contribute to hyperglycemia.

***Fluid replacement*** must account for both blood loss and third-space loss:

- Blood: Replacement may be with lactated Ringer's (3 mL to 1 mL blood loss) or 5% albumin colloid (1 mL to 1 mL blood loss) to maintain hematocrit at predetermined adequate minimal level:
- Infants and neonates: more than 30% (may be as high as 40% to 50%).
- Older children: 20% to 26%.

Blood is replaced with packed red blood cells when the allowable blood loss threshold is exceeded.

***Allowable blood loss*** is calculated by the following formula based on the child's average hematocrit:

- Average hematocrit = (beginning hematocrit + minimum adequate hematocrit) ÷ 2.
- Allowable blood loss = [estimated blood loss × (beginning hematocrit – minimum adequate hematocrit)] ÷ average hematocrit.

Blood loss should be monitored carefully to determine when it exceeds the allowable blood loss.

***Volume of packed red blood cell replacement*** is based on the hematocrit of packed cells, 75%:

- Packed red blood cells in mL = [(estimated blood loss – allowable blood loss) × minimum adequate hematocrit] ÷ packed red blood cell hematocrit of 75.

If blood loss exceeds 1 to 2 blood volumes, then 10 to 15 mL/kg of platelets and fresh frozen plasma (FFP) are administered.

**Third space loss** can only be estimated on the basis of the degree of trauma related to the surgery:

- Minor: 3-4 mL/kg/hr.
- Moderate: 5-6 mL/kg/hr.
- Severe: 7-10 mL/kg/hr.

Lactated Ringer's is most commonly used to replace third-space loss.

### Pediatric pharmacology

Volatile anesthetics

Small infants have higher water content (70%-75%) than adults (50%-60%) and a lower muscle mass. These factors, coupled with slow renal and hepatic clearance, increased rate of metabolism, decreased protein binding, and increased organ perfusion affect the **pharmacological action of**

**drugs.** Pediatric doses are calculated according to the child's weight in kilograms, but other factors may affect dosage. Weight is estimated by age (although actual weight is safer):

- 50th percentile weight (kg) = (Age × 2) + 9.

**Anesthetic agents** must be chosen with care because of the potential for adverse effects:

***Inhalational***: Infants are more likely to experience hypotension and bradycardia with inhalational anesthetic agents. Inhalation induction is rapid because infants and young children have higher alveolar ventilation and lower functional residual capacity (FRC) than older patients, and depression of ventilation is more common in infants. There is increased risk of overdose. Sevoflurane is usually preferred for induction, and isoflurane or halothane is preferred for maintenance, because desflurane and sevoflurane are associated with delirium on emergence.

Nonvolatile anesthetics
Pediatric **anesthetic agents** include the following:

***Nonvolatile***: Infants and small children may need higher proportionate (based on weight) doses of propofol because they eliminate it more quickly adults do. Propofol should not be used for children who are critically ill because it has been correlated with a higher mortality rate and severe adverse effects leading to multiorgan failure. Thiopental also is used in higher proportionate doses for infants and children but not for neonates. Neonates are especially sensitive to opioids, and morphine should be avoided or used with caution. The clearance rates of some drugs (sufentanil, alfentanil) may be higher in children. Ketamine combined with fentanyl may cause more hypotension in neonates and small infants than ketamine combined with midazolam. Midazolam combined with fentanyl can cause severe hypotension. Etomidate is reserved for children older than 10 years.

Muscle relaxants
Pediatric **anesthetic agents** include the following:

***Muscle relaxants:*** Onset with muscle relaxants is about 50% shorter in infants and children than in adults, and pediatric patients may have variable responses to nondepolarizing muscle relaxants. Drugs that are metabolized through the liver (pancuronium, vecuronium, and cisatracurium) have prolonged action; therefore, atracurium and cisatracurium, which do not depend on the liver, are more reliable. Because succinylcholine can cause severe adverse effects (rhabdomyolysis, malignant hyperthermia, hyperkalemia, arrhythmias), its use requires premedication with atropine, but succinylcholine is usually avoided in pediatric patients except for rapid sequence induction for children with full stomach and laryngospasm. Rocuronium is frequently used for intubation because of fast onset, but its duration is up to 90 minutes; therefore, mivacurium, atracurium, and cisatracurium may be preferred for shorter procedures. Nerve stimulators should be used to monitor incremental doses, which are usually 25% to 30% of the original bolus. Blockade by nondepolarizing muscle relaxants can be reversed with neostigmine or edrophonium and glycopyrrolate or atropine.

## Pediatric anesthesia techniques and procedures

<u>Preoperative considerations</u>

A number of **preoperative considerations** are important in preparing a pediatric patient for surgery:

- ***Preparing the child:*** Children are often very frightened of pain and separation from parents; therefore, the anesthetist should take the time to show children the equipment (such as masks) and explain the procedure in terms suited for the child's age. If possible, a parent or caregiver may be allowed to stay with the children during induction.
- ***Health considerations:*** Children with viral upper respiratory infections have increased pulmonary complications with surgery (wheezing, laryngospasm, hypoxemia, and atelectasis). Thus, surgery may be delayed, especially if the child is febrile, or anticholinergic agents may be given preoperatively and mask ventilation may be used with humidification of inspired gas to reduce irritation.
- ***Laboratory review:*** Requirements for preoperative laboratory studies vary from one institution to another. Some centers require no laboratory tests for healthy children undergoing minor surgery; in such cases, careful evaluation is necessary to determine which children require laboratory testing and which tests are appropriate.
- ***Food and fluid restriction:*** Because small children are more likely to become dehydrated, restrictions are less strict than for older children and adults. Infants less than 6 months old are given formula or breast milk up to 4 hours before surgery and clear liquids until 2 to 3 hours before surgery. Infants aged 6 to 36 months are given formula or breast milk and solids up to 6 hours before surgery and clear fluids until 2 to 3 hours before surgery.
- ***Premedication:*** There is no real consensus about the best premedication, and neonates and infants who are ill are usually not premedicated, however, premedication with midazolam has been proven to decrease anxiety in children as compared to placebo/parent presence. Atropine is often given to prevent hypotension and bradycardia during induction and to prevent secretions, especially with upper urinary tract infection. Atropine may be given orally or with the IV before induction. There is a lower rate of negative post op behaviors in children who receive premedication.

## Pediatric anesthesia techniques and procedures

<u>Monitoring</u>

**Monitoring**, as for adults, must be adjusted for pediatric limits. Pulse oximetry and capnography are monitored carefully for hypoxia. In neonates, the pulse oximeter is usually placed on the right hand or earlobe. End-tidal $CO_2$ analysis is less reliable in infants because of tachypnea and small tidal volumes. Core temperature must be monitored carefully because of increased risk of hypothermia and malignant hyperthermia. Invasive monitoring must be performed with great care so that air embolism can be avoided, and pulmonary artery catheterization is usually avoided. Children who are likely to suffer hypoglycemia (those receiving hyperalimentation or those born of diabetic mothers) should be monitored for serum glucose concentration. Arterial or central venous catheters may be used for blood sampling in pediatric patients who are critically ill or if blood loss is beyond allowable limits, requiring transfusion.

<u>IV access and intraosseous (IO) infusion</u>

**IV access** can be difficult to establish in neonates and infants younger than 2 years. The saphenous vein in the ankle is often accessible. Care must be taken to eliminate all air bubbles so that air embolism can be prevented.

**Intraosseous (IO) infusion** is an alternative to IV access for neonates and pediatric emergencies when rapid access is necessary or when peripheral or vascular access cannot be achieved. It is often used in cases of pediatric cardiac arrest. Because yellow marrow replaces red marrow, establishing access in patients older than 5 is more difficult. Preferred sites include the following:

- 0-5 years: Proximal tibia (preferred).
- Older children and adults: medial malleolus. The sternum can support higher infusion rates. Other sites include the distal femur, clavicle, humerus, and ileum.

IO infusion is used for administering fluids and anesthesia and for obtaining blood samples. Equipment requires a special needle (13-20 gauge) because standard needles may bend. The bone injection gun (BIG) with a loaded spring facilitates insertion. Position is confirmed by aspiration of blood and marrow.

## Induction and maintenance

**Induction** in pediatric patients can be achieved with IV or inhalational anesthetics. IV induction is usually used if the child arrives in the operating room with an existing IV; it includes a rapid-acting barbiturate, such as thiopental or propofol, and then a nondepolarizing muscle relaxant, such as atracurium, cisatracurium, mivacurium, rocuronium, or succinylcholine (with atropine given before succinylcholine). If no IV is in place, children are often given nitrous oxide (70%) and oxygen (30%), sometimes with insufflation over the face or a clear mask to allay fears. Alternately, sevoflurane 7% to 8% in 60% nitrous oxide may be used for faster induction. Sevoflurane or halothane are typically added in 0.5 increments every 3-5 breaths. **Maintenance** is similar to that for adults, usually with isoflurane or halothane. An opioid (fentanyl) may be used 15 to 20 minutes before the end of surgery if sevoflurane is used for maintenance; the opioid will reduce tremors and agitation during emergence. Ventilation must be carefully controlled, and care must be taken not to deliver large tidal volumes.

## Pediatric complications management

### Laryngospasm

**Laryngospasm:** This brief spasm of the larynx (vocal cords) is a common complication of pediatric surgery. Laryngospasm is caused by stimulation of the superior laryngeal nerve and may occur any time during surgery, although it is most common during extubation or in the immediate postoperative period. Extubation while the patient is deeply anesthetized (before cough or swallowing reflexes have return) when the patient is awake decreases incidence of laryngospasm. Children who have been exposed to environmental tobacco smoke are at approximately 10 times greater risk of laryngospasm than those not exposed. Treatment includes jaw thrust, IV lidocaine, or nondepolarizing muscle relaxants, such as succinylcholine or rocuronium. Children should be positioned in the lateral position during recovery so that secretions do not pool about the vocal cords.

### Postintubation croup and pain

**Postintubation croup:** This condition is caused by edema of the glottis or trachea and usually occurs within 3 hours after surgery. Care must be taken to selecting a correctly sized ETT so that irritation can be prevented. IV dexamethasone may be given as prophylaxis, but if edema occurs, inhalation of nebulized racemic epinephrine is used as treatment.

**Pain:** At one time it was believed that small infants did not feel pain, but this belief is no longer considered true. Infants and children should be provided with adequate analgesia. This may consist of regional analgesia, such as peripheral nerve blocks, spinal anesthesia, epidurals, and caudal

- 89 -

blocks (usually with lidocaine or bupivacaine and morphine sulfate or hydromorphone). Less-invasive treatment includes acetaminophen suppositories and parenteral opioids, such as fentanyl, morphine, hydromorphone, and meperidine. Patient-controlled analgesia (PCA) may be used for children aged 6 years or older (depending on maturity), usually with a 10-minute lockout and morphine or hydromorphone (which may also be used for continuous infusions).

## Congenital anomalies

### Hirschsprung's disease

**Hirschsprung's disease:** a congenital disorder causing infants to be born without intestinal ganglion nerve cells in part or all of the colon, resulting in mechanical obstruction. The disease may be an acute life-threatening condition or a chronic condition. Normally, nerves signal the colon to contract, pushing the stool through the colon, but the absence of propulsion in the segments without ganglions causes the fecal material to accumulate. Affected areas almost always include the rectum and distal colon, but in rare instances the disease can "skip" segments and involve the entire colon, including the small intestine. As fecal material collects, the segment of the bowel proximal to the defect distends, creating megacolon. The internal rectal sphincter may fail to relax as well, preventing evacuation and contributing to obstruction. Hirschsprung disease accounts for approximately 25% of all neonatal obstructions, is 4 times more common in boys than in girls, may have a genetic link, and is more common in infants with Down syndrome.

### Malrotation and omphalocele

**Malrotation**: Occurring during fetal development, this condition causes an abnormality in the rotation and fixation of the midgut area, resulting in omphalocele, umbilical hernia, gastroschisis, congenital diaphragmatic hernia, or mesocolic paraduodenal hernia.

**Omphalocele** is a congenital herniation of the intestines or other organs through the base of umbilicus with a protecting amniotic membrane but no skin. The sac may contain only a loop or most of the bowel and the internal abdominal organs. Diagnosis is usually made by fetal ultrasonography. Symptoms vary widely. Maintaining the integrity of tissues by keeping the exposed sac or viscera moist and providing intravenous fluids is important. Small omphaloceles are repaired immediately, but more extensive repair is usually delayed until infant's condition is stable if the sac is intact. Silvadene cream toughens the sac, which is usually covered with a silastic (plastic) pouch. The abdomen may be unusually small, making correction difficult; therefore, surgeons may delay the correction for 6 to 12 months while the abdominal cavity grows. Surgical repair may be performed in stages over a period of 8 to 10 days.

### Imperforate anus

**Imperforate anus (anorectal malfunction)** is a congenital abnormality in which the rectum is absent, malformed, or displaced from its normal position. Imperforate anus may include disorders of the urinary tract. It occurs in 1 in 5000 births, more commonly in boys than in girls. Imperforate anus may include stenosis or atresia of the anus. There are 3 main categories, classified according to the relationship of the rectum to the puborectalis musculature:

- *Low anomalies:* No external opening, but the rectum is otherwise in normal position through the puborectalis muscle, with normal function, and has no connection to the genitourinary tract.
- *Intermediate anomalies:* Rectum is at or below the level of the puborectalis muscle, and an anal dimple is evident. The external sphincter is in the normal position.

- *High anomalies:* Rectum ends above the puborectalis muscles, and the internal sphincter is absent. Frequently, there is a rectourethral fistula in boys or a rectovaginal fistula in girls. There may be fistulas to the bladder or perineum.

## Epispadias, hypospadias, and posterior urethral valves

**Epispadias** is a condition in which the urethral orifice is in an abnormal position and the pubic bone is widened. In boys, the urethra may open on the top (dorsum), the sides, or the complete length of the penis; in girls, the urethra, with a urethral cleft along its length, usually bifurcates the clitoris and labia but may be in the abdomen. Boys may have a short, wide penis with abnormal chordee (curvature). The condition is 3 to 5 times more common among boys than among girls.

**Hypospadias** is a condition in which the urethral orifice opens onto the ventral surface of the penis. The diagnosis is made by physical examination and endoscopy to evaluate the bladder neck and the external sphincter. Intravenous pyelography evaluates the urinary tract. Symptoms include urinary incontinence, infections, and reflux nephropathy (backward flow of urine to kidneys).

**Posterior urethral valves:** a urethral abnormality in boys in which urethral valves have narrow, slit-like openings that impede urinary flow and allow reverse flow that can damage the urinary organs, which swell and become engorged with urine.

## Persistent cloaca, cloacal exstrophy, bladder exstrophy, and ureteropelvic junction obstruction

**Persistent cloaca:** a condition in girls in which there is an imperforate anus and the rectum, vagina, and urethra form a single channel with a rectal fistula attached to the posterior wall of the channel.

**Cloacal exstrophy:** a rare and complicated disorder of the pelvic area that usually includes multiple abnormalities of the intestinal, urinary, and reproductive systems as well as skeletal abnormalities.

**Bladder exstrophy:** an eversion of the posterior wall of the bladder through the anterior wall of the bladder and through the lower abdominal wall, with the bladder and urethra exposed, a wide pubic arch, anterior displacement of the anus, and abnormalities of the reproductive organs.

**Ureteropelvic junction obstruction (UPI):** a congenital obstruction at the point at which the ureter connects to the renal pelvis, unilaterally or bilaterally, causing inadequate urinary flow and hydronephrosis. This condition improves markedly in some infants within the first 18 months, but others require surgery.

## Pulmonary agenesis and aplasia

**Pulmonary agenesis** is the complete absence of the carina (the ridge formed by the lowest tracheal cartilage between the right and left bronchi), bronchus, lung, and vasculature. **Pulmonary aplasia** is absence of the lung and vasculature, but the carina and partial bronchus are present. Bilateral conditions are inconsistent with life but are very rare; unilateral agenesis or aplasia is often associated with skeletal, cardiac, or other anomalies (in 50% of cases). Lobar agenesis may occur, but it is less common than absence of the entire lung. Pulmonary agenesis or aplasia is usually diagnosed in childhood but can easily be overlooked, even with chest radiography. The condition, if not accompanied by other anomalies, is often essentially asymptomatic unless the remaining lung is compromised by disease or infection. There is no treatment, because the lung is missing, but preventive measures include the following:

- Aggressive treatment of infections.
- Precautions during general anesthesia because of inadequate respiratory reserve.

## Congenital diaphragmatic hernia and respiratory distress

**Congenital diaphragmatic hernias (CDHs)** may cause severe respiratory distress. The primary CDHs that affect children are posterolateral (Bochdalek):

- Left-sided CDH (85% of cases) includes herniation of the large and small intestine and intraabdominal organs into the thoracic cavity.
- Right-sided CDH (13% of cases) may be asymptomatic; usually only the liver and part of the large intestine herniate.

Neonates with left-sided CDH may exhibit severe respiratory distress and cyanosis. The lungs may be underdeveloped because of pressure exerted from displaced organs during fetal development. There may be a left hemothorax with a mediastinal shift, and the heart may press on the right lung, which may be hypoplastic. Bowel sounds are heard over the chest area. Pulmonary hypertension and cardiopulmonary failure may occur. Despite treatment, mortality rates are 50%, and children who survive may have emphysema, with larger volume but inadequate numbers of alveoli.

## Inborn errors of metabolism

**Inborn errors of metabolism** comprise a wide range of genetic metabolic disorders, usually related to defects in gene coding for enzymes, resulting in toxic accumulations that interfere with metabolism. Disorders are classified according to the type of metabolic disorder and include the following:

- *Carbohydrate* (glycogen storage disease, fructose intolerance)
- *Proteins* (clotting defects, sickle cell anemia, thalassemia, osteogenesis imperfecta, Marfan syndrome)
- *Amino acids* (phenylketonuria, hyperammonemia)
- *Organic acid* (alcaptonuria)
- *Cholesterol/lipoprotein* (hyperlipoproteinemias, hypoproteinemia)
- *Mitochondrial* (Kearns-Sayre syndrome)
- *Porphyrin* (porphyria)
- *Defective DNA repair* (xeroderma pigmentosum)

Symptoms relate to the specific defect. Some symptoms are present in the neonate; others appear in childhood or adulthood. Some diseases are life-threatening, and others are slowly progressive. Manifestations common to many disorders may include encephalopathy with poor feeding, lethargy, tachypnea, metabolic acidosis or hyperammonemia (or both), hypoglycemia, hepatic dysfunctions with jaundice, dysmorphism (structural anomalies), and abnormal body odor or urine odor.

<u>Pulmonary lobar emphysema, bronchogenic cysts, pulmonary cysts, cystic adenomatoid</u>
<u>malformation, and pulmonary sequestration</u>

There are a number of congenital pulmonary anomalies:

- *Congenital lobar emphysema* occurs when one lobe is over-expanded, compressing the other lobes and causing a mediastinal shift.
- *Bronchogenic cysts* originate from the tracheobronchial tree; they are usually round and can cause significant compression, depending on their size.
- *Pulmonary cysts* occur within the parenchyma of the lungs, generally in a single lower lobe. Larger cysts or small cysts that begin to expand can result in respiratory compromise.
- *Cystic adenomatoid malformation (CAM)* is a thoracic hamartoma (benign tumor-like nodule resulting from an overgrowth of mature cells and tissue in the affected part). Overgrowth of bronchioles and alveoli is common, ranging from cystic-type masses to solid, nodular masses.
- *Pulmonary sequestration* is an unusual mass of primitive tissue that is found inside (intralobar/intrapulmonary) or outside (extrapulmonary) the lung tissue but does not communicate with the tracheobronchial tree.

## Congenital neurological abnormalities

<u>Myelomeningocele</u>

**Myelomeningocele,** which involves spina bifida cystica with a meningeal sac containing spinal fluid and part of the spinal cord and nerves, accounts for approximately 75% of the total cases of spina bifida. There are numerous physical manifestations.

- *Exposed sac* poses the danger of infection and cerebrospinal fluid leakage. Surgical repair is usually performed within the first 48 hours after birth, although it may be delayed for a few days, especially if the sac is intact.
- *Chiari type II* malformation consists of hypoplasia of the cerebellum and displacement of the lower brainstem into the upper cervical area, which impairs the circulation of spinal fluid. It may result in symptoms of cranial nerve dysfunction (dysphonia, dysphagia) and in weakness and lack of coordination of upper extremities.
- *Neurogenic bladder* is common and may require the Credé maneuver for infants and, later, intermittent clean catheterization.
- *Fecal incontinence* is common; as the child ages, it is controlled by diet and bowel training.
- *Musculoskeletal abnormalities* depend on the level of the myelomeningocele and the degree of impairment but often involve the muscles and joints of the lower extremities and sometimes the upper extremities. Dysfunction often increases with the number of shunts. Scoliosis and lumbar lordosis are common. Hip contractures may cause dislocations.
- *Paralysis or paresis* may vary considerably and be spastic or flaccid. Many children require wheelchairs for mobility, although some are fitted with braces that assist ambulation.
- *Seizures* occur in approximately 25% of affected children, sometimes related to shunt malfunction.
- *Hydrocephalus* is present in approximately 25% to 35% of infants at birth and in 60% to 70% after surgical repair with ventriculoperitoneal shunt. Untreated, the ventricles will dilate and brain damage can occur.
- *Tethered spinal cord* occurs when the distal end of the spinal cord becomes attached to the bone or the site of surgical repair and does not move superiorly with growth, causing increased pain, spasticity, and disability, and requiring surgical repair.

<u>Spina bifida</u>

The terms **spina bifida** and **myelomeningocele** are often used interchangeably, but there is a distinction. Spina bifida is a neural tube defect with an incomplete spinal cord and often missing vertebrae that allow the meninges and spinal cord to protrude through the opening. There are 5 basic types:

- ***Spina bifida***: A defect in which the vertebral column is not closed, with varying degrees of herniation through the opening.
- ***Spina bifida occulta***: Failure of the vertebral column to close, but because there is no herniation through the opening, the defect may not be obvious.
- ***Spina bifida cystica***: Defect in closure, with external sac-like protrusion and varying degrees of nerve involvement.
- ***Meningocele***: Spina bifida cystica with a meningeal sac filled with spinal fluid.
- ***Myelomeningocele***: Spina bifida cystica with a meningeal sac containing spinal fluid and part of the spinal cord and nerves.

<u>Down syndrome (trisomy 21)</u>

**Down syndrome** (trisomy 21) is a congenital disease that occurs as a result of a trisomy (3 copies) of chromosome 21 or 14; 21 unbalanced translocation. There are a number of clinical manifestations:

- ***Dysmorphism:*** Small skull with flat occiput, inner epicanthal folds, an upward and outward slant to eyes, saddle nose, protruding tongue, highly arched palate, short and thick neck, hypotonic musculature, lax joints, Simian line on palm, and broad, short, stubby hands and feet.
- ***Intellectual impairment:*** May range from mild to profound retardation.
- ***Range of congenital anomalies:*** Congenital heart disease, renal agenesis, duodenal atresia, Hirschsprung disease, tracheoesophageal fistula, hip subluxation, and instability of cervical vertebrae 1 and 2.
- ***Sensory deficits:*** Hearing loss, strabismus, nystagmus, cataracts, conjunctivitis, and myopia.
- ***Growth impairment:*** Reduced height and weight and delayed sexual development.

# Obstetrics

## Obstetric anatomy, physiology, and pathophysiology

<u>Labor and delivery important factors</u>

A number of interrelated factors are crucial for successful **labor and delivery**:

- ***Birth passage:*** The size of the pelvis, type of pelvis (shape), and ability of the cervix to dilate and efface and the vagina and introitus to distend.
- ***Fetus:*** The size of the fetal head, the attitude (flexion or extension, with flexion the normal attitude), the lie in relationship to the maternal spine (longitudinal, more than 99%; transverse, less than 1%; transverse leads to complications), and presentation (cephalic most common) during descent. Additional factors include the molding ability of the skull at the sutures (frontal, sagittal, coronal, and lambdoidal).
- ***Fetal/birth passage relationship:*** Engagement of fetal presenting body part, station in the maternal pelvis, and position in the maternal pelvis.
- ***Force of labor:*** Effectiveness of uterine contractions (frequency, duration, intensity) and effectiveness of maternal pushing efforts.

- **Psychological and social issues:** Preparation for childbirth (psychological and physical), values and beliefs, previous pregnancies and deliveries, family/partner/spousal support, and emotional status.

## Uterine blood flow

**Uterine blood flow** is a crucial factor in the viability of the fetus. Uterine blood flow is estimated as the following:

- Uterine arterial pressure – venous pressure / uterine vascular resistance.

During pregnancy, uterine vessels dilate and uterine blood flow increases from about 50 mL/min to 700 mL/min to supply the placenta (80%) and myometrium (20%). Because of the extensive vessel dilation, autoregulation is absent; therefore, factors that decrease uterine arterial pressure, increase venous pressure, or increase arterial resistance can impede uterine blood flow and result in fetal distress. These conditions include hypotension, vasoconstriction, contractions of the uterus, stress (which triggers catecholamines), $\alpha$-adrenergic agonists (used for hypotension), vasopressors (phenylephrine), seizures, aortocaval or venocaval compression, and $Paco_2$ lower than 20 mm Hg. Ephedrine is usually used to treat hypotension because it controls blood pressure without interfering with uterine blood flow.

## Obstetric pharmacology

### Placental transfer of drugs

The **placenta** acts as a barrier to protect the fetus, but its main function is to provide oxygen and nutrients for the fetus by linking the maternal and fetal circulation. Virtually all **drugs** cross the barrier to some degree, some by active transport. Some drugs are readily diffused across the placental barrier and can affect the fetus. Drugs that are non-ionized, fat-soluble, and of low molecular weight diffuse easily, as does glucose. Once a substance crosses the barrier, the lower pH of the fetal blood allows weakly basic drugs, such as local anesthetics and opioids, to cross into the fetal circulation where they become ionized and accumulate because they cannot pass back into the maternal circulation (ion trapping). Giving an intravenous injection during a contraction, when uterine blood flow decreases, reduces the amount of the drug that crosses the placental barrier. A few drugs with large molecules (heparin, insulin) have minimal transfer, and lipid-soluble drugs transfer more readily than water-soluble drugs.

### Opioids and sedatives

**Opioids and sedatives** are usually given only in the early stages of labor, because they readily cross the placental barrier and can cause central nervous system depression in the fetus. This depression can persist after delivery, especially in premature infants, and can affect Apgar scores. Some drugs, such as morphine and benzodiazepines, are avoided because of excessive fetal depression. IV PCA pumps are being used with less risks, better pain relief, and greater patient satisfaction. Common opioids being used include the following:

- Meperidine (1-25 mg IV or 25-50 mg IM to a maximum of 100 mg) is the most common dose. IV onset is 1 to 20 minutes and IM onset is 1 to 3 hours. Meperidine use is limited to more than 4 hours before delivery.
- Fentanyl (25-100 µg/hr IV) has shorter onset (3-10 minutes) with 1 hour duration and causes less fetal depression.

- Butorphanol 1-2 mg or nalbuphine 10-20 mg IV or IM causes few respiratory effects and provides adequate relief of pain but may result in excessive sedation if given repeatedly.
- Promethazine (25-50 mg IM) and hydroxyzine may be used in combination with meperidine or alone to provide relief of anxiety and to reduce the opioid dose.

## Cesarean section with regional anesthesia

**Cesarean sections** are performed if there is increased risk of uterine rupture, maternal hemorrhage, and dystocia including fetal-pelvic disproportion and breech presentation, and emergent situations, such as fetal distress or impending maternal death.

**Regional anesthesia** (spinal, epidural) is associated with lower mortality rates than general anesthesia and is the preferred anesthetic approach. Additionally, there is less fetal depression, a reduced risk of maternal pulmonary aspiration, and an opportunity to provide neuraxial analgesia for postoperative pain relief. Regional anesthesia must provide a T4 sensory level, which causes a high sympathetic blockade. This should be treated with 1000 to 1500 mL of Ringer's lactate before spinal blockade and 500 mL for epidural. One hour before blockade, the patient should be given 15 to 30 mL sodium citrate (oral antacid). The patient receives the regional anesthesia and is then placed in supine position (slight Trendelenburg to facilitate blockade) with left uterine displacement.

Blood pressure must be constantly monitored and IV ephedrine 10 mg given if necessary to prevent hypotension, because systolic BP lower than 95 mm Hg may cause decreased uterine blood flow, and systolic BP lower than 100 mm Hg for 10 to 15 minutes may cause fetal acidosis and bradycardia. Supplemental oxygen is administered at 40% to 50%:

- ***Spinal:*** A hyperbaric solution of tetracaine, lidocaine, or bupivacaine is injected with the patient in sitting or lateral decubitus position. Epinephrine may be added to enhance block, and opioids (fentanyl or sufentanil) may be added to prolong duration of block and provide postoperative analgesia.
- ***Epidural:*** Lidocaine 2% (with or without epinephrine) or chloroprocaine 3% is usually administered via epidural catheter. Sodium bicarbonate may be added to increase speed of onset, and opioids (fentanyl or sufentanil) may be added to prolong and enhance blockade. Anesthetic agents are given in incremental doses to maintain adequate analgesia. Opioids may be continued after surgery for pain relief. The larger doses for epidural may be absorbed systemically and cross the placenta, affecting the fetus.

## Cesarean section with general anesthesia

In some cases, **general anesthesia** may be administered for **Cesarean section,** although because the risks to the mother are intensified, general anesthesia is usually limited to emergent situations in which the mother or the fetus is at risk:

- Fetal distress during 2nd stage of labor.
- Tetanic uterine contractions.
- Patient confused and uncontrollable and unable to cooperate (such as psychiatric patients).
- Inverted uterus.
- Retained placenta.
- Breech extraction or other position requiring version and extraction.

- 96 -

The mother is placed supine with left uterine displacement (wedge under left hip) to avoid pressure on the inferior vena cava or aorta; such pressure can result in hypotension. Sodium citrate (0.5-1 oz) is given 1 hour before surgery, and the mother is preoxygenated for 3 to 5 minutes or hyperventilated with approximately 5 deep breaths before rapid-sequence induction with cricoid pressure (propofol 2 mg/kg or thiopental 3-4 mg/kg and succinylcholine 80-100 mg). A nondepolarizing NMBA is not generally needed to prevent fasciculations, which are usually prevented by increased levels of progesterone.

Tracheal tube placement should be verified by capnography before skin incision, because inability to ventilate during surgery is the primary cause of maternal death. After induction, maintenance is by 50% nitrous oxide/50% oxygen with a small dose of volatile anesthetic (1-2 MAC concentration) in 100% $O_2$, which is increased slightly before delivery to relax the uterus and then decreased again to less than 0.5 MAC after delivery. A medium-duration muscle relaxant is given. An oxytocin infusion (20-30 U/L IV fluids) is started. An opioid and nitrous oxide or propofol may be administered after the delivery is complete to provide amnesia and prevent recall. If the mother was nonfasting or if aspiration is a concern, an orogastric tube may be inserted for aspiration of stomach contents to reduce the chance of aspiration during emergence. Additionally, the patient should be extubated only after awake. Blood loss with Caesarean section is about 1000 mL; therefore, fluid replacement must balance estimated loss.

## Vaginal delivery

### First stage of labor and delivery
The stages of labor differ somewhat from one woman to another and in multipara and nullipara:

**First stage:** This stage signals onset of labor with regular contractions and proceeds until the cervix is fully dilated. There are 3 phases:

- **Latent**: This early phase may persist for 8.5 hours for nullipara and 5.3 hours for multipara. The cervix begins to dilate (≤3 cm), and contractions may occur every 3 to 30 minutes, lasting for 20 to 40 seconds. The intensity of the contractions is usually mild to moderate (25-40 mm Hg as measured by an intrauterine pressure catheter, IUPC). The mother is usually able to cope with discomfort and may feel some anxiety.
- **Active**: This phase may persist for 4.5 hrs in the nullipara and 2.5 hours in the multipara. The cervix dilates to 4 to 7 cm (1.2 cm/hr for nullipara and 1.5 cm/hr for multipara) with contractions increasing in frequency every 1 to 5 minutes, lasting for 40 to 60 seconds. The intensity is moderate to strong (50-70 mm Hg per IUPC), and anxiety and pain increase.
- **Transition**: This phase may persist for 3.6 hours for the nullipara and approximately 1 hour for the multipara, although the duration may increase by an hour with epidural anesthesia. The cervix becomes fully dilated to 8 to 10 cm with frequent contractions every 1.5 to 2 minutes, lasting for 60 to 90 seconds. The intensity is strong by palpation and 70 to 90 mm Hg per IUPC. During this stage, the mother may experience much anxiety and pain and the feeling that bearing down or contractions will tear her apart. Cervical dilation slows to between 8 to 10 cm, and fetal descent increases (1 cm/hr for nullipara and 2 cm/hr for multipara). Mothers frequently request pain medication and may hyperventilate, have difficulty following directions, cry or moan, become very restless, hiccup, belch or vomit, and complain of rectal pressure.

## Second stage of labor and delivery

The **second stage of labor** begins when the cervix is fully dilated and ends with delivery. This stage usually lasts for about 2 hours for the nullipara and only 15 minutes for the multipara. Frequent contractions continue every 1.5 to 2 minutes and last for 60 to 90 seconds (as in the transition phases of stage 1), and intensity is very strong by palpation and 70 to 100 mm Hg by IUPC. As the fetal head descends, it applies pressure to the sacral and obturator nerves, causing an intense urge to bear down. The perineum begins to bulge and flatten out, and bloody show increases. The mother often feels severe pain and burning in the perineal area. The fetal head crowns as delivery is imminent. The perineum thins as the fetal head distends the vulva and the anus, sometimes causing stool to be expelled. The head is born, followed by the shoulders and body in a spontaneous (non-breech) birth.

## Third and fourth stages of labor and delivery

The **third stage of labor** commences after the delivery of the infant and ends after the placenta is delivered. After delivery, strong uterine contractions decrease the surface area of the placental attachment, causing separation, which is accompanied by bleeding and formation of a hematoma between the decidua and the placental tissue. Finally, the placental membrane peels off of the uterine wall. Signs of placental separation usually occur between 5 and 30 minutes after birth:

- Globular-shaped uterus.
- Fundus rises in the abdomen.
- Increased gush or trickling of blood.
- Umbilical cord protrudes farther from the vagina.

A placenta is considered retained if it has not separated more than 30 minutes after delivery.

The **fourth stage** extends from 1 to 4 hours after birth, during which the mother's body goes through physiologic readjustment. Blood is redistributed and this, coupled with a blood loss of 250 to 400 mL, contributes to moderate hypotension and tachycardia. The uterus stays contracted, and the fundus is usually midline between the symphysis pubis and the umbilicus.

## Pudendal nerve block

Visceral pain occurs during the first stage of labor from contractions and cervical dilation with afferent impulses entering the spinal cord at T10-T11. However, during the second stage of labor, the stretching of the vagina and perineum caused by descent of the fetus causes somatic pain with impulses carried by the pudendal nerves to the spinal cord at S2-S4. **Pudendal nerve block** is used during the second stage (sometimes along with perineal infiltration) to reduce somatic pain when neuraxial blocks are contraindicated and for episiotomy and relaxation of the pelvic floor for forceps delivery. With the patient in lithotomy position, a transvaginal or transperineal approach is used to block the nerve. For the transvaginal approach (the most common), a Kobach needle or special guide (Iowa trumpet) is used to prevent inadvertent injection into the fetal head. Anesthetic agents include 10 mL of 1% lidocaine or 2% chloroprocaine. The transperineal approach may be used if the head is engaged.

## Lumbar epidurals

The most common form of regional anesthesia or analgesia for labor and delivery is the **lumbar epidural**. Dilute mixtures of local anesthetic and opioids are combined. The catheter is usually placed early so that it is in place when pain relief is needed. At one time, epidurals were delayed until labor was well established, but current trends are to administer them earlier if the fetus is in no distress, contractions are 3 to 4 minutes apart and persisting for at least 60 seconds, and the fetal head is engaged with 3 to 4 cm of cervical dilation. The catheter is usually placed with the mother in the sitting position to ensure sacral spread. Placement is usually at L3-L4 or L4-L5. If inadvertent spinal placement occurs, spinal anesthesia or analgesia may be given or the catheter may be removed and replaced at a higher level. Most commonly, bupivacaine or ropivacaine (0.0625%-0.125%) is given in combination with fentanyl (2-3 μg/mL) or sufentanil (0.3-0.5 μg/mL). If dilute anesthetic agents are used, the mother may be able to ambulate while receiving the epidural.

For activation during the ***first stage of labor***, IV fluid (500-1000 mL) with lactated Ringer's is administered during placement of the epidural catheter. Glucose-containing fluids are avoided because they may cause maternal hyperglycemia and neonatal hypoglycemia as a result of increased secretion of insulin in response to the glucose. A test dose of 3 mL local anesthetic (usually lidocaine 1.5%) is given to verify correct catheter placement. If placement is correct, the patient is placed in the supine position and 10 mL of opioid-anesthetic mixture is administered in 2 doses 1 to 2 minutes apart and repeated as needed throughout the first stage. For activation during the ***second stage***, procedures are similar, with injection between contractions. After a test dose, the opioid-anesthetic mixture is given with 10 to 15 mL at no more than 5 mL every 1 to 2 minutes. Oxygen is given and the patient is placed in the supine position with left uterine displacement and monitoring of BP every 1 to 2 minutes for 15 minutes and then every 5 minutes. Combined spinal/epidural may be used for severe pain.

### Spinal anesthesia (saddle block)

A **saddle block**, or spinal anesthesia, is usually given just before vaginal delivery to provide rapid perineal anesthesia. Spinal blocks are avoided during labor because they interfere with motor function. Because of this, other agents may be used during labor. Before receiving spinal anesthesia, the patient is given a bolus of 500 to 1000 mL fluid. With the patient in a sitting position, a very small spinal needle (to prevent CSF leakage and postspinal headache) is inserted into the subarachnoid space. Local anesthetics used include hyperbaric tetracaine, bupivacaine, and lidocaine, often with the addition of fentanyl or sufentanil to potentiate the effect. The agents are administered between contractions over about 30 seconds. The patient remains seated for 3 minutes and then is placed in the lithotomy position with left uterine displacement to prepare for delivery.

### Intrathecal analgesia with opioids

**Intrathecal analgesia** with **opioids** alone is sometimes used during the first stage of labor. Commonly used agents include morphine (0.25-0.5 mg), meperidine (10-15 mg), fentanyl (12.5-15 μg), and sufentanil (2-10 μg). Meperidine is the only agent that has local anesthetic characteristics. Higher doses are needed if spinal opioids are used alone, administered as a single dose or intermittently per catheter, and this can result in a higher risk of complications, maternal respiratory depression, and fetal depression. However, if given alone, opioids (except for meperidine) do not provide motor blockade or maternal hypotension; therefore, the mother is able to push. However, the analgesic effect may not be adequate, and adverse effects related to the agent may occur, such as pruritus, nausea, and vomiting. Morphine alone has a slow onset (45-60 minutes) although it provides 4 to 6 hours of analgesia with spinal administration, but low doses may not provide adequate relief and high doses increase adverse effects. Morphine is frequently combined with fentanyl for more rapid onset. Commonly, opioids are combined with local anesthetics.

### Epidural analgesia with opioids

**Epidural analgesia** with **opioids** alone is also sometimes used during the first stage of labor. Commonly used agents include morphine (5 mg), meperidine (50-100 mg), fentanyl (50-150 µg), and sufentanil (10-20 µg). The duration of analgesia is longer with epidural administration of opioids than with intrathecal, but many of the same problems occur. Low doses of morphine may not provide adequate pain relief, and higher doses may cause respiratory depression. Morphine has a slow onset (0.5 to 1 hour) but provides analgesia for 12 to 24 hours. Meperidine provides good relief but is short-acting (1 to 3 hours). Fentanyl and sufentanil both have rapid onset but are also short acting (1 to 2 hours). Commonly, morphine is combined with fentanyl or sufentanil for fast onset with long duration. The fetus must be monitored carefully if repeated epidural doses of opioids are administered because they can cause fetal depression.

### Postpartum tubal ligation

**Postpartum tubal ligation** may be performed immediately after cesarean, delayed for 8 to 48 hours after vaginal delivery, or performed 6 weeks after delivery, depending on the circumstances. Concerns after general anesthesia include the danger of aspiration with prolonging anesthesia. Some physicians prefer to perform the ligation after a period of fasting. If an epidural was used for vaginal labor and delivery, the epidural can be left in place for as long as 48 hours; this delay ensures that the woman is fasting and that she will not change her mind after delivery. If the delivery occurred without anesthesia, a regional (preferred) or general anesthetic may be administered for tubal ligation. Spinal anesthesia is often preferred rather than epidural because it obviates the risk of inadvertent IV or intrathecal injection of epidural anesthetics. Tetracaine or lidocaine is used for spinals, and lidocaine or chloroprocaine is used for epidurals. If laparoscopic tubal fulguration is chosen, it is delayed for 6 weeks and is generally performed with the patient under general endotracheal anesthesia because insufflation impairs gas exchange.

### Vaginal birth after Cesarean section

There has been decreasing interest in **vaginal birth after Cesarean section**; only 10% of patients have attempted it in recent years. However, many mothers can undergo vaginal delivery without complications. Risks include hemorrhage and uterine rupture (1%). Women who attempt vaginal birth have a 60% to 80% success rate. Guidelines for vaginal delivery after Cesarean include the following:

- Candidates: A woman who has undergone one previous Cesarean delivery using a low transverse uterine incision should be advised to attempt vaginal birth. A woman who has undergone 2 or more previous Cesarean sections may attempt vaginal births.
- In all cases, a physician, an anesthesiologist, and adequate staff must be present and available throughout labor to provide a Cesarean section if necessary.

Contraindications to attempting vaginal delivery include T or classic incision, history of myomectomy, contracted pelvis, obstetrical complications precluding vaginal birth, and inadequate facilities or staff to provide emergency Cesarean section if it is needed.

## High risk (diabetes)

**Maternal diabetes mellitus** poses increased risks for both the mother and the fetus. Most risks relate to hyperglycemia, so strict control of glucose levels (70-120 mg/dL) is critical:

- *Maternal risks* include hydramnios related to excessive fetal urination, preeclampsia/eclampsia if there are diabetes-related vascular changes, hyperglycemia, and ketoacidosis, which can lead to maternal coma and death or fetal death. Fetal-pelvic disproportion related to fetal macrosomia may result in dystocia (difficult labor). Mothers may experience worsening of retinopathy.
- *Fetal risks* include congenital anomalies (5%-10%), macrosomia (which may cause birth trauma with vaginal delivery), intrauterine growth restriction, respiratory distress syndrome, hyperbilirubinemia, and hypocalcemia.

Regional anesthesia during delivery can reduce uterine blood flow. Pudendal block with small doses of opioids may be used or continuous epidural may be administered if there is no fetal distress. Regional blockade during Cesarean may cause cardiovascular depression; therefore, preloading with dextrose-free IV is necessary. Glucose monitoring must be performed throughout general anesthesia, because the epinephrine response to decreasing glucose levels is decreased.

## High risk (older mothers)

**Older mothers** (older than 35 years) have a higher risk of miscarriage (>50% by age 42) and fetal abnormalities, but if they are in good health, there is little evidence that they are at higher risk during labor and delivery. Problems arise if pregnancy is associated with other health problems, such as hypertension or diabetes, and older mothers are at increased risk of both of these conditions for the first time during pregnancy. Older mothers have a higher rate of Cesarean section; factors that contribute to this hither rate are slower onset and progression of labor, with prolongation of the second stage of labor, and the administration of oxytocin. Fetal distress is also more common. Studies have shown that Cesarean rates among older mothers do not necessarily correlate with complications; this finding suggests that Cesarean may be used as an elective procedure or as a precaution. Anesthetic management is similar to that for younger mothers.

## High risk (preeclampsia)

A diagnosis of preeclampsia includes blood pressure ≥140/90 mm Hg with an onset after twenty weeks' gestation and proteinuria >300 mg/24hr. Seizures are a major complication of preeclampsia, and magnesium sulfate is the drug of choice for preventing seizures in this patient population. Magnesium sulfate therapeutic range is 4-8 mEq/L, and increased levels lead to widening of the QRS complex, a prolonged QT interval, SA block, paralysis, and arrest. Deep tendon reflexes should be frequently checked on patients receiving magnesium sulfate. This drug increases sensitivity to nondepolarizing muscle relaxants. Mag toxicity is treated with IV calcium. While high blood pressure should be treated, it should not be normalized. Placental blood flow is proportionate to maternal blood pressures, so sudden and large changes in blood pressure could be compromising for the fetus. The most commonly used antihypertensive agent in preeclampsia is hydralazine, due to few effects on uterine blood flow. Patients with refractory hypertension, severe cardiac disease, severe pulmonary disease, refractory oliguria, and pulmonary edema should have invasive central monitoring during anesthesia.

### Non-obstetric surgery in the parturient

**Non-obstetric surgery** occurs in about 1% to 2% of pregnancies. The most common procedures are laparoscopy, appendectomy, and cholecystectomy. Surgery poses an increased risk for both the mother and the fetus because hypovolemia, hypotension, anemia, hypoxemia, and sympathetic activation may interfere with the transfer of oxygen and nutrients across the placental barrier. Exposure to anesthetic agents should be minimized. In the first two weeks of pregnancy, drugs may have lethal or no effect, but the greatest risk occurs during weeks 3 through 8, because this is when organs develop. After the 8th week, physiological abnormalities and growth deficits may occur. The safest period is after 20 to 24 weeks of gestation, especially with regional anesthesia rather than general. Spinal anesthesia results in less maternal and fetal drug exposure than epidural, although general anesthesia may be preferred for some procedures, such as cholecystectomy. Fetal heart rate and uterine activity must be monitored along with standard monitoring of the mother. In rare cases, cardiopulmonary bypass (CPB) has been used for critical procedures, but arrest of circulation should be avoided.

# Geriatrics

### Cardiovascular system

A number of physiological changes associated with aging may affect **geriatric** anesthesia:

- *Cardiovascular system:* Patients may have existing heart disease, such as CHG, coronary artery disease, or hypertension that predisposes them to a decrease in arterial elasticity with increased systolic blood pressure and afterload. Left ventricular hypertrophy is common. Baroceptor response decreases. Marked diastolic dysfunction may be present. Both resting and maximal heart rates may be reduced, making it more difficult for the body to respond to conditions that require increased oxygen, such as hypovolemia, hypotension, and hypoxia. Enlargement of the atria correlates with atrial fibrillation and flutter and development of congestive heart failure (CHF). Patients may suffer from hypotension during induction because of decreased cardiac reserve. Reduced cardiac output causes a prolonged circulation time. Onset of IV drugs may be delayed because of slower circulation time, but onset of inhalational anesthesia may be faster.

### Metabolic/endocrine, renal, and hepatic systems

Many systems are affected in **geriatric** patients:

- *Metabolic/endocrine system:* Thermoregulation is less stable; therefore, hypothermia and malignant hyperthermia may occur more readily. Production of heat decreases and heat loss increases, and the temperature-regulating mechanism of the hypothalamus may reset internal temperature control at a lower level. Because insulin resistance tends to increase, there is less ability to handle glucose.
- *Renal system:* As cardiac output decreases, renal blood flow also decreases along with a decrease in the glomerular filtration rate (about 6% to 8% each decade) and decreased tubular length. There is also some impairment of sodium balance, concentrating and diluting, and water conservation ability. These problems may cause fluid overload or dehydration; therefore, urinary output should be maintained at 0.5 mL/kg/hr, and anesthetic agents that are cleared through the kidneys must be monitored carefully.
- *Hepatic system:* Liver mass and liver blood flow decrease with age; therefore, clearance of drugs through the liver is slowed, and less albumin is produced.

## Pulmonary system

There are a number of respiratory considerations in **geriatric** patients:

- *Pulmonary system:* Common diseases of the pulmonary system include emphysema, COPD, chronic bronchitis, and pneumonia. Typically, aging patients exhibit decreases in pulmonary elasticity, decreases in alveolar surface area with alveolar distention, decreases in residual volume, and decreases in arterial oxygen tension with increased closing capacity, ventilation/perfusion mismatching, and chest wall rigidity, which impairs the exchange of oxygen. Because overall strength is often decreased, there is less ability to breathe deeply and to cough. Diminished protective laryngeal reflexes result in a greater chance of aspiration; therefore, a cuffed endotracheal tube (ETT) should be used with cricoid pressure during induction. The minimal alveolar concentration (MAC) of inhalational anesthetics is decreased. Extended preoxygenation before induction and increased concentration of oxygen during surgery are needed for preventing hypoxia. Those with preexisting respiratory diseases and those who have undergone major abdominal surgery are often left intubated postoperatively. Regional and neuraxial blocks may be considered to control pain and facilitate pulmonary function.

## Pharmacology and anesthetic requirements (inhalational)

**Pharmacological considerations** related to the numerous changes associated with aging affect both the drug dose and the plasma concentration of drugs. In general, anesthetic requirements are decreased and the effects of anesthetics are prolonged; therefore, short-acting agents, such as propofol, desflurane, remifentanil, and succinylcholine are frequently preferred. Other drugs may be chosen because they are less dependent on the liver or kidneys for clearance (atracurium, cisatracurium, and mivacurium). Anesthetic considerations include the following:

- *Inhalational*: The minimal alveolar concentration of these drugs decreases by approximately 4% each decade (after the age of 40). Drugs that depress cardiac function have an exaggerated effect, and those that cause tachycardia are attenuated. Recovery is often prolonged. Because desflurane is eliminated rapidly, it is often preferred for the elderly. Another agent frequently used is isoflurane, which decreases vascular resistance but has little effect on cardiac output and causes less tachycardia than in younger patients. It has rapid onset and short duration.

## Nervous, musculoskeletal, and immune systems

Additional systems affected in **geriatric** patients:

- *Nervous system:* Brain mass tends to decrease with age, corresponding to a loss of neurons (especially in the frontal lobes) and decreased cerebral blood flow. Short-term memory loss is most common, but mentation usually remains intact unless there is an underlying disorder, such as Alzheimer disease or stroke. The effects of general anesthesia tend to be prolonged with a lower dosage requirement, and many elderly people experience postoperative cognitive dysfunction (POCD), which may persist for weeks or months and may occasionally be permanent. Postoperative delirium can occur with both regional and general anesthesia. Peripheral nerve cells may degenerate, causing muscle atrophy. The threshold for sensory input may increase.
- *Musculoskeletal system*: Vessels become fragile, muscle mass decreases, fat content increases, and joints may become stiff, limiting mobility.

- ***Immune system:*** The elderly often have decreased antibody-mediated and cell-mediated immune responses, leaving them less able to combat infections. Fever response to inflammation and infection may be impaired.

## Pharmacology and anesthetic requirements

<u>Nonvolatile and muscle relaxants</u>

A number of **pharmacological** considerations are associated with other anesthetic agents:

- ***Nonvolatile***: Elderly patients require lower doses of many nonvolatile anesthetic agents, including propofol, etomidate, opioids, barbiturates, and benzodiazepines. Dosage requirements for all of these drugs may be as much as 50% less than for young adults, depending on the patient's age.
- ***Muscle relaxants***: Onset of neuromuscular blockade may be prolonged with decreased cardiac output. The action of drugs that are cleared through the liver (rocuronium, vecuronium) or kidneys (metocurine, pancuronium, doxacurium, and tubocurarine) may be prolonged. Drugs that are not affected by aging include atracurium and pipecuronium. Succinylcholine is prolonged in men (lower levels of plasma cholinesterase) but not in women.
- ***Neuraxial anesthetics***: Spinal anesthesia is prolonged. Epidural anesthetics have increased cephalad spread and provide a shorter duration of analgesia and motor block.

## Geriatric surgery complications

Geriatric surgery poses an increased risk of **complications**, but there has been a steady decrease in morbidity and mortality related to surgical procedures over the past few decades with better anesthetic management and understanding of the special needs of geriatric patients. Complications and mortality rates are higher with emergency procedures than with elective procedures, but this is true for patients in all age groups. This finding suggests that delaying surgery in the elderly is counterproductive if the result may be an emergency operation. Factors that contribute to increased complications include the number of coexisting morbidities and poor nutritional status. Congestive heart failure and neurologic history are associated with increased pulmonary complications. Recent studies have shown that chronological age alone poses much less risk than other factors, such as illness. Postoperative cognitive deficit (POCD) can occur in elderly patients regardless of the surgical anesthetic agent used, although duration of anesthetic, pulmonary complications, history of neurological disease, second operation, and infections all appear to contribute to this outcome. POCD is associated with increased mortality so preventive steps should be taken to minimize it including using limiting medications associated with delirium in the elderly, preventing hypoxemia and hypercarbia, and providing sufficient postoperative analgesia.

# Professional Issues

### Leadership and accountability

Nurse anesthetists, especially those in leadership positions, have a responsibility to assist others with **professional leadership and accountability** within the healthcare team and the community. Collaboration requires an ongoing commitment that includes mentoring, coaching, and teaching others. Anesthetists must be involved in the following:

- Making decisions at all levels of an organization or facility.
- Taking an active role in strategic planning.
- Assuming responsibility for standards of surgical care.
- Assessing and selecting equipment and supplies and electronic equipment, including information systems.
- Assisting in planning for utilization of resources.
- Analyzing all decisions with respect for patient outcomes.
- Supporting staff education and development, including training for management positions and opportunities for acquiring continuing education hours.
- Facilitating access to research and to both internal and external resources.
- Allowing staff members the time to consider their place in the organization and their own practice.

### Negligence

Risk management attempts to determine the burden of proof for acts of **negligence**, including compliance with duty, breaches in procedures, degree of harm, and cause. Negligence indicates that *proper care* has not been provided, according to established standards. *Reasonable care* uses a rationale for decision-making in relation to providing care. State regulations regarding negligence may vary, but all have some statutes of limitation. There are a number of different types of negligence:

- ***Negligent conduct*** indicates that a person failed to provide reasonable care or to protect or assist another, according to standards and expertise.
- ***Gross negligence*** is the willful provision of inadequate care with disregard of the safety and security of another.
- ***Contributory negligence*** occurs when the injured party contributes to his or her own harm.
- ***Comparative negligence*** requires a determination of the percentage amount of negligence that is attributed to each person involved.

### Professional liability

Professional liability is defined by risk management to ensure that related risks are minimized. Direct providers of care must obtain consents for medical care, provide adequate care, and obey drug laws. Physicians may have liability for a wide range of issues, including misdiagnosing, failing to supervise other staff, providing incorrect or substandard treatment, treating patients outside area of expertise, failing to provide follow-up care, failing to seek necessary consultation, infections resulting from procedures, premature discharge, and lack of proper documentation. Anesthetists may also be liable for improperly administering drugs or anesthesia, failing to follow standard medical procedures, failing to follow physician's orders or to take correct oral or verbal orders, and failing to report changes in a patient's conditions or defective equipment.

## Interdisciplinary collaboration

**Interdisciplinary collaboration** is absolutely crucial to medical practice if the needs and best interests of the patients and families are central. Interdisciplinary practice begins with the nurse anesthetist and surgeon but extends to pharmacists, social workers, occupational and physical therapists, nutritionists, and a wide range of allied healthcare providers, all of whom cooperate in diagnosis and treatment. However, state regulations determine to some degree how much autonomy a nurse anesthetist can have in diagnosing and treating. Although nurses, in general, have increasingly gained more legal rights, they have also become more dependent on collaboration with others for their expertise and for referrals if the patient's needs extend beyond the nurse's ability to provide assistance. Additionally, the prescriptive ability of nurse anesthetists varies from state to state; some states require direct supervision by other professionals (such as physicians), whereas others require particular types of supervisory arrangements, depending on the circumstances.

## Quality improvement models

### Juran's QIP

Joseph **Juran's quality improvement process (QIP)** is a 4-step method, focusing on quality control, that is based on a trilogy of concepts: quality planning, control, and improvement. The steps of the QIP process are the following:

- *Defining* the project involves organizing; listing and prioritizing problems; and identifying a team.
- *Diagnosing* involves analyzing problems, using root cause analysis to formulate theories, and testing theories.
- *Remediating* includes considering various alternative solutions and then designing and implementing specific solutions and controls while addressing institutional resistance to change. As causes of problems are identified and remediation is instituted to remove the problems, the processes should improve.
- *Holding* involves evaluating performance and monitoring the control system so that gains can be maintained.

### PDCA

**Plan-Do-Check-Act (PDCA)** (Shewhart cycle) is a method of continuous quality improvement. PDCA is simple and understandable; however, consistently maintaining this cycle may be difficult because of lack of focus and commitment. PDCA may be more suited to solving specific problems than organization-wide problems:

- *Plan*: identifying, analyzing, and defining the problem, setting goals, and establishing a process that coordinates with leadership. Extensive brainstorming, including fishbone diagrams, identifies problematic processes and lists current process steps. Data are collected and analyzed, and a root cause analysis is completed.
- *Do*: Generating solutions, selecting one or more of them, and implementing the solution on a trial basis.

- *Check*: Gathering and analyzing data to determine the effectiveness of the solution. If it is effective, then continue to *Act*; if not, return to *Plan* and pick a different solution. (*Study* may replace *Check: PDSA.*)
- *Act*: Identifying changes that are necessary for fully implementing the solution, adopting the solution, and continuing to monitor results while selecting another improvement project.

## Quality improvement

### Financial issues

Performance improvement is not without costs, and these must be considered carefully in cost analysis. **Financial costs related to quality** management include the following:

- ***Error-free costs*** are all those costs in terms of processes, services, equipment, time, materials, and staffing that are necessary for providing a product or process that is without error from the onset. A process that is error free is relatively stable in terms of preestablished guidelines.
- ***Cost of quality*** (COQ) includes costs associated with identifying and correcting errors, making errors, defects or failures in processes and planning, and costs of poor quality (COPQ). Conformance costs are those costs related to preventing errors, such as monitoring and evaluation. This may include education, maintenance, pilot testing, and analysis. Nonconformance costs are those related to errors, failures, and defects. These may include adverse events (such as infections), poor access because of staff shortages or cancellations, lost time, duplications of service, and malpractice.

### American Health Information Management Association's process improvement model

The American Health Information Management Association's **process improvement model** for performance improvement is a consensus-building method with 11 steps:

1. Create a list of opportunities for improvement through brainstorming, and prioritize the list, choosing one on which to focus.
2. Define the project and create the quality improvement team that will facilitate the improvement process.
3. Analyze problems related to the process.
4. Create a speculative list of causes as a beginning point.
5. Test assumptions.
6. Perform root cause analysis to identify specific causes related to problems.
7. Consider a number of alternative solutions.
8. Design possible solutions and controls.
9. Reach consensus by addressing resistance to change through education, inservice, and presentations.
10. Implement solutions and controls.
11. Evaluate performance.

## Professional practice standards

<u>AANA Code of Ethics</u>

The **American Association of Nurse Anesthetists** (AANA) has established a **Code of Ethics** for the CRNA, and each member must adhere to the standards. The Code establishes that CRNAs practice in accordance with responsibilities outlined by the state, the nursing profession, and society:

1. ***Responsibility to patients:*** The CRNA must provide quality anesthesia care while protecting the moral and legal rights and safety of the patient and ensuring that informed consent has been obtained. The CRNA must not exploit or abuse a relationship of trust with the patient. The CRNA must provide care regardless of national or ethnic background, sex, age, religious preference, disability, and social or economic background. The CRNA may withdraw from providing care only because of personal convictions if no harm comes to the patient and if such refusal is not a breach of duty.
2. ***Competence***: The CRNA must maintain an RN license, recertify as a CRNA as required, and participate in lifelong education and quality improvement practices.
3. ***Professional Responsibilities:*** The CRNA collaborates with others to promote the profession and is responsible for personal judgment and actions related to professional practice.
4. ***Societal Responsibilities:*** The CRNA collaborates with those in the community and others in healthcare professions to promote community and national efforts to provide for the public's health needs.
5. ***Product/Service Endorsement:*** Endorsements must be truthful, non-exploitive, and based on personal experience. They must not claim AANA endorsement unless the Board of the AANA has made an endorsement.
6. ***Research***: The CRNA conducts research, participates in research, and ensures that research follows ethical and reporting standards, protecting rights and wellbeing of research subjects, both human and animal.
7. ***Business Practice:*** Ethical business practices must be consistent with professional standards.

<u>Documenting record of anesthesia</u>

The American Association of Nurse Anesthetists has issued a Standard of Care for documenting the Record of Anesthesia:

- Patient identifying information, including physical information necessary to providing anesthesia: weight, height, sex, allergies, physical condition.
- Anesthesia provider: This includes first anesthetist, second anesthetist, and any relief staff (including the person's credentials and the times the person provided relief).
- Safety check of equipment according to established protocol to ensure that equipment is functioning.
- Outline of monitoring (minimal standards): ECG, BP, precordial stethoscope, pulse oximetry, $O_2$ analyzer, end-tidal $CO_2$.
- Outline of graphic monitoring display (minimal standards): ECG, BP, heart rate, ventilation status, $O_2$ saturation.
- Additional monitoring depending on procedures and needs: Esophageal stethoscope; thermometer; nerve stimulators; respirometers; arterial, central venous, and pulmonary artery catheters and lines; and EEG.

- 108 -

- Graphic or other recording of monitoring information, depending on the type of monitoring; for example, if a ventilator is used, information includes tidal/minute volume, peak inspiratory pressure, and rate. If temperature is monitored, the readings must be documented. (Continued)
- Airway management includes documenting the specific mask and intubation used, whether intubation was performed with the patient awake or asleep, techniques, difficulties, and assessment of ETT placement (and method of ensuring placement, such as breath sounds, $ETco_2$ reading), method of securing tube, method of inflating tube, times of intubation and extubation, ventilation parameters, and use of nasal or oral airway.
- Medications used must include name, dosage, administration route, time, total dosage, and adverse reactions.
- Anesthesia technique includes types of anesthetic agents used for induction and maintenance, location and size of IVs, identification of all monitoring lines, techniques used for regional anesthesia, and results.
- Intake includes all blood, crystalloids, colloids, volume expanders, and other products.
- Output includes urine, blood loss, drainage per tubes, such as NG, and ascites.
- Process includes date, procedure, starting and stopping time (24-hour clock).
- Patient protection includes position, changes, and protective measures for body parts (such as eye protection) and securing of lines and ETT.

## Patient safety

### Medical errors

Assessment of patient safety must include a consideration of **medical errors,** unintentional but preventable mistakes in providing care. *Errors* are classified as failures to carry out a planned action or the use of the wrong plan, whereas an *adverse event* is the negative result of that error, such as an injury:

- Errors may result from commission (doing something) or omission (failing to do something).
- Errors can be active, resulting from contact between the patient and an aspect of the medical system, such as a nurse or piece of equipment.
- Errors can be latent, resulting from a failure of design in the system.
- Error chains are the series of events that lead to a negative outcome, usually identified by root cause analysis.

Medical errors are most often identified after an adverse event occurs, but some may not be identified and are found on medical record reviews.

### External factors

The patient safety culture is constantly evolving in response to new information, technology, and both internal and external forces. A number of **important external forces** affect the development of an organization's patient safety culture:

- External regulations or legislation and healthcare initiatives, such as state and federal laws and Leapfrog, promote and mandate safe practices that can improve patient safety and provide optimal cost-effective care.

- Accreditation agencies provide mandates and standards for healthcare organizations and their leaders that can reduce risk and improve patient safety. For example, the Joint Commission has issued the National Practice Safety Guides (NPSG) to assist healthcare organizations in assessing and developing safe practices.
- Professional organizations, such as the American Association of Nurse Anesthetists, have principles and codes of ethics that require quality care and patient safety.

## Facilitating safe passage

Facilitating **safe passage** is part of caring practice that ensures patient safety, in a broad sense, from a variety of perspectives:

- Giving appropriate medications and treatment without errors that endanger the patient's health is essential.
- Providing information to the patient and family about treatments, changes, conditions, and other aspects related to care helps them to cope with the situations as they arise.
- Preventing infection is central to patient safety and includes the use by staff of proper infection-control methods, such as handwashing.
- Knowing the patient requires the nurse to take the time and effort to understand the needs and wishes of the patient and family.

Assisting with transitions involves helping the patient and family cope not only with moving from one form of treatment or one unit to another but also with transitions in health, such as from illness to health or from illness to death.

## Anesthesia errors

The nurse anesthetist must always provide diligence to avoid **anesthesia errors.** The most common errors involve the following:

- Inappropriate dosage of medication or anesthesia.
- Delay in onset of anesthesia because of equipment malfunction, dosing errors, or other complications.
- Incorrect or traumatic intubation that causes respiratory distress, obstruction, or injury.
- Inadequate monitoring before, during, and after surgery.
- Improper treatment or complications, failure to recognize complications, or neglect of complications.
- Leaving the patient unattended during surgery.
- Improper administration of oxygen.
- Use of or failure to report use of drugs or alcohol by those involved in the surgical procedure.
- Excessive sedation that prolongs anesthesia.
- Improperly cared for or defective anesthesia equipment.
- Anesthesia awareness, in which the patient remains aware during the procedure, hearing conversations, feeling respiratory distress, or feeling pain.

# CRNA Practice Test

*Note: The length of the review material in this document indicates the broad scope of the CRNA test content. These questions provide four answer choices for each question.*

1. Which of the following is not a side effect of the cholinoreceptor blocker atropine?

   a. Increased pulse
   b. Urinary retention
   c. Constipation
   d. Mydriasis

2. Which of the following is not a side effect of the ACE inhibitor captopril?

   a. Rash
   b. Angioedema
   c. Cough
   d. Congestion

3. Which of the following is not a side effect of the vasodilator nifedipine?

   a. Nausea
   b. Flush appearance
   c. Vertigo
   d. Sexual dysfunction

4. Which of the following is not a side effect of the sympathoplegic clonidine?

   a. Hypertension
   b. Asthma
   c. Dry oral cavity
   d. Lethargic behavior

5. Which of the following is not a side effect of loop diuretics?

   a. Alkalosis
   b. Nausea
   c. Hypotension
   d. Potassium deficits

6. Which of the following is not an effect of isoflurane?

   a. Elevated lipid levels
   b. Nausea
   c. Increased blood flow to the brain
   d. Decreased respiratory function

7. Which of the following is not an effect of midazolam?

   a. Amnesia
   b. Decreased respiratory function
   c. Anesthetic
   d. Dizziness

8. Which of the following is not an effect of clozapine?

    a. Agranulocytosis
    b. Antipsychotic
    c. Used for schizophrenia
    d. Increased appetite

9. Which of the following is not treated with epinephrine?

    a. Renal disease
    b. Asthma
    c. Hypotension
    d. Glaucoma

10. Which of the following is not treated with ephedrine?

    a. COPD
    b. Hypotension
    c. Congestion
    d. Incontinence

11. Which of the following are not treated with barbiturates?

    a. Seizures
    b. Hypotension
    c. Insomnia
    d. Anxiety

12. Which of the following are not treated with opioid analgesics like dextromethorphan and methadone?

    a. Pulmonary edema
    b. Cough suppression
    c. Sedation
    d. Pain

13. Which of the following are not treated with hydrochlorothiazide?

    a. CHF
    b. Hypertension
    c. Nephritis
    d. Hypercalciuria

14. Which of the following are not treated with nifedipine?

    a. Angina
    b. Arrhythmias
    c. Hypertension
    d. Fluid retention

15. Which of the following is not treated with methotrexate?

    a. Sarcomas
    b. Leukemias
    c. Ectopic pregnancy
    d. Rheumatic fever

16. Which of the following are not treated with prednisone?

    a. Cushing disease
    b. Testicular cancer
    c. Lymphomas
    d. Chronic leukemias

17. Which of the following are not treated with dexamethasone?

    a. Inflammation
    b. Asthma
    c. Addison's disease
    d. Wilson disease

18. Which of the following are not treated with lansoprazole?

    a. Zollinger-Ellison syndrome
    b. Gastritis
    c. Hypertension
    d. Reflux

19. Which of the following is the antidote for the toxin heparin?

    a. Protamine
    b. Methylene blue
    c. N-acetylcysteine
    d. Glucagon

20. Which of the following is the antidote for the toxin copper?

    a. Glucagon
    b. Aminocaproic acid
    c. Atropine
    d. Penicillamine

21. Which of the following is the antidote for the toxin benzodiazepines?

    a. Flumazenil
    b. Methylene blue
    c. Deferoxamine
    d. Alkalinize urine

22. Which of the following is the antidote for the toxin lead?

    a. Naloxone
    b. Nitrite
    c. Calcium EDTA
    d. Dialysis

23. Which of the following is the primary site of activity for warfarin?

    a. Kidney
    b. Liver
    c. Blood
    d. Heart

24. Lansoprazole is not used in which of the following cases?

    a. Gastritis
    b. Peptic ulcers
    c. Zollinger-Ellison syndrome
    d. Thalamus hypertrophy

25. Which of the following drugs is associated with the reaction of cinchonism?

    a. Valproic acid
    b. Quinidine
    c. Isoniazid
    d. Ethosuximide

26. Which of the following drugs is associated with the reaction of hepatitis?

    a. Valproic acid
    b. Quinidine
    c. Isoniazid
    d. Ethosuximide

27. Which of the following drugs is associated with the reaction of Stevens-Johnson syndrome?

    a. Valproic acid
    b. Quinidine
    c. Isoniazid
    d. Ethosuximide

28. Which of the following drugs is associated with the reaction of tendon dysfunction?

    a. Digitalis
    b. Niacin
    c. Tetracycline
    d. Fluoroquinolones

29. A drug ending in the suffix (pril) is considered a _____.

    a. $H_2$ agonist
    b. ACE inhibitor
    c. Antifungal
    d. Beta agonist

30. A drug ending in the suffix (azole) is considered a _____.

    a. $H_2$ agonist
    b. ACE inhibitor
    c. Antifungal
    d. Beta agonist

31. A drug ending in the suffix (tidine) is considered a _____.

    a. Antidepressant
    b. Protease inhibitor
    c. Beta antagonist
    d. $H_2$ antagonist

32. A drug ending in the suffix (navir) is considered a _____.

    a. Antidepressant
    b. Protease inhibitor
    c. Beta antagonist
    d. $H_2$ antagonist

33. Which of the following drugs is associated with the reaction of extreme photosensitivity?

    a. Digitalis
    b. Niacin
    c. Tetracycline
    d. Fluoroquinolones

34. Which of the following is not related to drug toxicity of prednisone?

    a. Cataracts
    b. Hypotension
    c. Psychosis
    d. Acne

35. Which of the following is not related to a drug toxicity of atenolol?

    a. Congestive heart failure (CHF)
    b. Tachycardia
    c. AV block
    d. Sedative appearance

36. Which of the following is considered a class IA sodium channel blocker?

    a. Mexiletine
    b. Amiodarone
    c. Quinidine
    d. Procainamide

37. Which of the following is considered a class IA sodium channel blocker?

    a. Propafenone
    b. Disopyramide
    c. Amiodarone
    d. Quinidine

38. Potassium-sparing diuretics have the primary effect upon the ____ found in the kidney.

    a. Proximal convoluted tubule
    b. Loop of Henle
    c. Collecting duct
    d. Distal convoluted tubule

39. Which of the following is not directly related to drug toxicity of nitroglycerin?

    a. Headaches
    b. Tachycardia
    c. Dizziness
    d. Projectile vomiting

40. Which of the following is not directly related to drug toxicity of ibuprofen?

    a. Nausea
    b. Renal dysfunction
    c. Anemia
    d. Muscle wasting

41. Which of the following drugs is a histamine blocker and reduces levels of gastric acid?

    a. Omeprazole (*Prilosec*)
    b. Metoclopramide (*Reglan*)
    c. Cimetidine (*Tagamet*)
    d. Magnesium hydroxide (*Maalox*)

42. Which of the following drugs is an antacid?

    a. Omeprazole (*Prilosec*)
    b. Metoclopramide (*Reglan*)
    c. Cimetidine (*Tagamet*)
    d. Magnesium hydroxide (*Maalox*)

43. Which of the following drugs is a dopamine antagonist?

    a. Omeprazole (*Prilosec*)
    b. Metoclopramide (*Reglan*)
    c. Cimetidine (*Tagamet*)
    d. Magnesium hydroxide (*Maalox*)

44. Which of the following is not considered an $H_2$ blocker?

    a. Ranitidine (*Zantac*)
    b. Famotidine (*Pepcid*)
    c. Cimetidine (*Tagamet*)
    d. Sucralfate (*Carafate*)

45. Which of the following drugs aids in gastric emptying?

    a. Cisapride (*Propulsid*)
    b. Ranitidine (*Zantac*)
    c. Famotidine (*Pepcid*)
    d. Tranylcypromine sulfate (*Parnate*)

46. Insulin inhibits the release of _____.

    a. Glucagon
    b. Antidiuretic hormone
    c. Beta cells
    d. Somatostatin

47. Which of the following is caused by insulin release?

    a. Increased breakdown of fats
    b. Increase breakdown of proteins
    c. Decreased blood sugar
    d. Causes glucose to be phosphorylated in kidney

48. Which of the following is not an adverse effect of glucagon?

    a. Allergic reaction
    b. Vomiting
    c. Nausea
    d. Fever

49. Which of the following is not generally caused by COPD?

    a. Pneumonia
    b. Right-sided heart failure
    c. Headaches
    d. Cor pulmonale

50. Which of the following is not considered a COPD-related disease?

    a. Bronchiectasis
    b. Bronchial asthma
    c. Bronchitis
    d. Bronchial hypotension

51. Which of the following is an expectorant?

    a. Acetylcysteine
    b. Guaifenesin
    c. Theophylline
    d. Epinephrine hydrochloride

52. Which of the following is a bronchodilator?

    a. Acetylcysteine
    b. Guaifenesin
    c. Theophylline
    d. Epinephrine hydrochloride

53. Which of the following is a xanthine?

    a. Acetylcysteine
    b. Guaifenesin
    c. Theophylline
    d. Epinephrine hydrochloride

54. Which of the following is a mucolytic?

    a. Acetylcysteine
    b. Guaifenesin
    c. Theophylline
    d. Epinephrine hydrochloride

55. Thyroid hormone $T_3$ does not have which of the following functions?

    a. Stimulate bone development and growth
    b. Create beta-adrenergic responses
    c. Cause brain development
    d. Decrease calcium reabsorption

56. Which of the following is not a function of estrogen?

    a. Causes breast growth
    b. Causes inhibition of follicle-stimulating hormone
    c. Increased follicle development
    d. Decreased overall transport proteins

57. A nurse anesthetist is reviewing a patient's medication. Which of the following medication would be contraindicated if the patient were pregnant? Note: More than one answer may be correct.

    a. *Coumadin*
    b. *Celebrex*
    c. *Catapres*
    d. *Habitrol*

58. A nurse anesthetist is reviewing a patient's past medical history. The history indicates photosensitive reactions to medications. Which of the following drugs has not been associated with photosensitive reactions? Note: More than one answer may be correct.

    a. *Cipro*
    b. Sulfonamide
    c. *Noroxin*
    d. *Nitro-Dur*

59. A patient tells you that her urine is starting to look discolored. If you believe this change is due to the patient's medication, which of the following does not cause urine discoloration?

    a. Sulfasalazine
    b. Levodopa
    c. Phenolphthalein
    d. Aspirin

60. A 34-year-old woman has recently been diagnosed with an autoimmune disease. She has also recently discovered that she is pregnant. Which of the following is the only immunoglobulin that will provide protection to the fetus in the womb?

    a. IgA
    b. IgD
    c. IgE
    d. IgG

61. *RhoGAM* is most often used to treat an ___ mother who has an ___ infant.

    a. RH positive, RH positive
    b. RH positive, RH negative
    c. RH negative, RH positive
    d. RH negative, RH negative

62. A nurse anesthetist is monitoring an infant who has recently been diagnosed with a congenital heart defect. Which of the following clinical signs would most likely be present?

    a. Slow pulse rate
    b. Weight gain
    c. Decreased systolic pressure
    d. Irregular WBC lab values

63. A patient's chart indicates a history of hyperkalemia. Which of the following would you not expect to see with this patient if this condition were acute?

    a. Decreased heart rate
    b. Paresthesia
    c. Muscle weakness of the extremities
    d. Migraines

64. A patient's chart indicates a history of ketoacidosis. Which of the following would you not expect to see with this patient if this condition were acute?

    a. Vomiting
    b. Extreme thirst
    c. Weight gain
    d. Acetone breathe smell

65. A patient's chart indicates a history of meningitis. Which of the following would you not expect to see with this patient if this condition were acute?

    a. Increased appetite
    b. Vomiting
    c. Fever
    d. Poor tolerance of light

66. A nurse anesthetist has a patient who has recently been diagnosed with renal failure. Which of the following clinical signs would most likely not be present?

    a. Hypotension
    b. Heart failure
    c. Dizziness
    d. Memory loss

67. A nurse anesthetist has a patient who has recently been diagnosed with hypokalemia. Which of the following clinical signs would most likely not be present?

    a. Leg cramps
    b. Respiratory distress
    c. Confusion
    d. Flaccid paralysis

68. A nurse anesthetist has a patient who has recently been diagnosed with metabolic acidosis. Which of the following clinical signs would most likely not be present?

    a. Weakness
    b. Dysrhythmias
    c. Dry skin
    d. Malaise

69. A nurse anesthetist has a patient who has recently been diagnosed with metabolic alkalosis. Which of the following clinical signs would most likely not be present?

    a. Vomiting
    b. Diarrhea
    c. Agitation
    d. Hyperventilation

70. A nurse anesthetist has a patient who has recently been diagnosed with respiratory acidosis. Which of the following clinical signs would most likely not be present?

a. $CO_2$ retention
b. Dyspnea
c. Headaches
d. Tachypnea

71. A nurse anesthetist has a patient who has recently been diagnosed with respiratory alkalosis. Which of the following clinical signs would most likely not be present?

a. Anxiety attacks
b. Dizziness
c. Hyperventilation cyanosis
d. Blurred vision

72. A nurse anesthetist is reviewing a patient's medication list. The drug pentoxifylline is present on the list. Which of the following conditions is commonly treated with this medication?

a. COPD
b. Coronary artery disease
c. Peripheral vascular disease
d. Multiple sclerosis

73. A patient has been on long-term management for CHF. Which of the following drugs is a loop diuretic that could be used to treat CHF symptoms?

a. Ciprofloxacin
b. Lepirudin
c. Naproxen
d. Bumetanide

74. A nurse anesthetist is reviewing a patient's medication. Which of the following is considered a potassium-sparing diuretic?

a. *Esidrix*
b. *Lasix*
c. *Aldactone*
d. *Edecrin*

75. A nurse anesthetist is reviewing a patient's medication. The patient is taking digoxin. Which of the following is not an effect of digoxin?

a. Depressed heart rate
b. Increased CO
c. Increased venous pressure
d. Increased contractility of cardiac muscle

76. A patient's chart indicates the patient is suffering from digoxin toxicity. Which of the following clinical signs is not associated with digoxin toxicity?

a. Ventricular bigeminy
b. Anorexia
c. Normal ventricular rhythm
d. Nausea

77. A patient has recently been diagnosed with hyponatremia. Which of the following is not associated with hyponatremia?

    a. Muscle twitching
    b. Anxiety
    c. Cyanosis
    d. Sticky mucous membranes

78. A patient has recently been diagnosed with hypernatremia. Which of the following is not associated with hypernatremia?

    a. Hypotension
    b. Tachycardia
    c. Pitting edema
    d. Weight gain

79. Which of the following blood therapeutic concentrations is abnormal?

    a. Phenobarbital, 10 to 40 mcg/mL
    b. Lithium, 4.2 to 9.7 mcg/mL
    c. Digoxin, 0.3 to 0.6 ng/mL
    d. Valproic acid, 40 to 100 mcg/mL

80. Which of the following blood therapeutic concentrations is abnormal?

    a. Triprolidine, 4 to 44 ng/mL
    b. Vancomycin, 30 to 40 mcg/mL
    c. Primidone, 0.2 to 1.9 mcg/mL
    d. Theophylline, 10 to 20 mcg/mL

81. Which of the following blood therapeutic concentrations is abnormal?

    a. Phenytoin, 10 to 20 mcg/mL
    b. Quinidine, 1 to 6 mcg/mL
    c. Haloperidol,6 to 245 ng/mL
    d. Carbamazepine, 15 to 25 mcg/mL

# Answer Key and Explanations

1. B: Although atropine blocks acetylcholine at the parasympathetic neuroeffector sites and will decrease GI and GU motility, its main job is to increase cardiac output and increase heart rate. Urinary retention is the least side effect to be expected.

2. D: Captopril decreases blood pressure and decreases preload and afterload in CHF, leading to an improvement in the symptoms of congestion.

3. D: Although sexual dysfunction may be a side effect for some patients, it is recognized as the least of the potential side effects from these selections.

4. A: Clonidine is given to patients with hypertension, as it is an alpha-agonist used to lower blood pressure. Hypertension therefore, is not a side effect of clonidine, but an indicator for its use.

5. B: Loop diuretics most often do not cause nausea. The other selections represent the most documented complaints from patients during clinical trials.

6. A: Isoflurane is a gas given as an anesthetic. It is given for a short amount of time and does not elevate lipid levels.

7. D: Midazolam (Versed) is used for its amnesia effect, as a preanesthetic medication, and it does lower respiratory rate. It may have the adverse effect of dizziness; it is not the drug of choice to treat for that symptom.

8. D: Clozapine is used to treat schizophrenia and as an antipsychotic. An effect of the drug is agranulocytosis and it is monitored by weekly or biweekly blood tests. Increased appetite is an adverse effect, which may lead to obesity.

9. A: Epinephrine may be used to treat asthma, low blood pressure, and glaucoma. It would not be the drug of choice in patients with renal disease.

10. A: Ephedrine could cause the symptoms of COPD to become more severe rather than improve. It is used to increase blood pressure, decrease nasal congestion, and improve incontinence caused by spasm.

11. B: Barbiturates lower blood pressure; they would not be used in the treatment of hypotension.

12. C: Dextromethorphan and methadone result in sedation because of their sedative effect. They would not be used to treat sedation.

13. C: Hydrochlorothiazide is a mild diuretic used in the management of CHF, hypertension, and hypercalciuria. It would not be used in the treatment of nephritis, inflammation of the kidney.

14. D: Nifedipine is used for cardiac conditions and may cause urinary symptoms. It is not given to treat fluid retention.

15. C: Methotrexate inhibits folic acid. It is given to help prevent the growth of malignant cells and for its immunosuppressive effects. It has no therapeutic use in ectopic pregnancy.

16. B: Prednisone may be given for its ability to suppress the migration of polymorph nuclear leukocytes and fibroblasts. It will decrease inflammation. It would not be helpful in testicular cancer.

17. D: Dexamethasone is used for asthma, allergies, and inflammation. It is contraindicated for renal diseases because it is excreted by the kidneys.

18. C: Lansoprazole decreases and suppresses gastric secretions and would have no therapeutic value in treating hypertension.

19. A: Protamine sulfate is given to treat an overdose of heparin. The other choices are specific to other conditions or symptoms.

20. D: Penicillamine is the antidote for copper toxicity.

21. A: Flumazenil (Mazicon) is given to counteract the effects of benzodiazepines by antagonizing the effects the drugs have on the CNS.

22. C: A level of lead greater than 45 mcg/dL in blood is treated with calcium EDTA, the chemical ethylenediaminetetraacetic acid.

23. B: Warfarin depresses hepatic synthesis of vitamin K, causing anticoagulant properties in the bloodstream.

24. D: Lansoprazole is used for decreasing gastric acids in conditions of the stomach. It would not be used to treat thalamus hypertrophy.

25. B: Quinidine will cause anachronism, tinnitus, and blurred vision.

26. C: Isoniazid is used to treat tuberculosis and is metabolized by the liver, increasing the risk of inflammation of the liver or hepatitis.

27. D: Ethosuximide (Zarontin) is associated with urticaria, pruritic erythema, and Stevens-Johnson syndrome.

28. D: Fluoroquinolones are broad-spectrum antibiotics that have been related to tendon toxicity in recent clinical studies.

29. B: Lisinopril is an example of an ACE inhibitor.

30. C: Antifungals are drugs most often ending in (azole). An example is itraconazole.

31. D: H2 antagonist medications most often end in (tidine) Ranitidine is an example of an H2 antagonist.

32. B: Protease inhibitors may end in (navir). An example of a protease inhibitor is saquinavir. These drugs are used to prevent and treat viral infections.

33. C: Tetracycline is associated with photosensitivity, which should be included in patient education.

34. B: Prednisone toxicity would cause hypertension.

35. B: Atenolol is used to treat supraventricular tachycardia; tachycardia is not related to the toxicity of the drug.

36. B: Amiodarone is considered a sodium channel blocker. Patients on this drug must have their electrolytes monitored frequently.

37. A: Propafenone is also a sodium channel blocker.

38. D: The distal convoluted tubule is located in the kidney and is the target area for potassium-sparing diuretics.

39. D: Projectile vomiting is not associated with nitroglycerin toxicity. The other choices are all symptoms of toxicity.

40. D: Muscle wasting is not a symptom of ibuprofen toxicity; however, nausea, renal dysfunction, and anemia may all be noted.

41. C: Cimetidine (Tagamet) is a histamine blocker and does reduce gastric acid. It may be prescribed for its histamine-blocking abilities in some cases of allergic reactions or asthma.

42. D: Maalox is the antacid.

43. B: Metoclopramide (Reglan) is a dopamine antagonist.

44. D: Sucralfate (Carafate) is considered an antiulcer or protectant and not an H2 blocker.

45. A: Propulsid was used to assist with gastric emptying before it was withdrawn from the market.

46. A: Glucagon is inhibited by insulin.

47. C: Insulin directly results in lower blood sugar levels.

48. D: Glucagon may cause an allergic reaction, vomiting, or nausea, but will not directly cause a fever.

49. C: COPD may increase the symptoms of or directly cause pneumonia and right-sided heart failure because of a decrease in the elasticity of the lungs. It has no direct relationship to headaches.

50. D: Bronchial hypotension would be the result of a vascular/cardiac problem and is not directly related to COPD.

51. B: Guaifenesin will help to loosen secretions so the patient can cough up the secretions.

52. D: Epinephrine hydrochloride is a bronchodilator. Theophylline is a spasmolytic.

53. C: Theophylline is in the chemical class xanthine.

54. A: Acetylcysteine is a mucolytic and in the chemical class of amino acid L-cysteine.

55. D: T3 does not decrease calcium reabsorption but increases it.

56. D: Estrogen does not decrease the transport of proteins.

57. A: Coumadin is the most significant drug listed if the patient is pregnant because it crosses the placenta.

58. D: Nitro-Dur has not been associated with photosensitivity. The other choices have been associated with photosensitivity.

59. D: Aspirin does not discolor urine.

60. D: IgG is the only protection for a fetus.

61. C: Rh- mothers are treated when the infant is Rh+ to protect the mother for other pregnancies and (+) antibodies.

62. B: Cardiac infants may have failure to gain weight but an abnormal weight gain indicates the infant has poor cardiac output.

63. D: Migraines are not associated with an increase in potassium. The other three selections are classic signs of hyperkalemia.

64. C: Patients with ketoacidosis most often have not been able to eat and have experienced a loss of weight due to illness and vomiting.

65. A: A patient with acute meningitis would have no appetite because of the symptoms of severe illness.

66. A: Acute renal failure most often is associated with hypertension.

67. D: Flaccid paralysis is not associated with hypokalemia.

68. B: Dysrhythmias may be associated with other disorders but the other selections would be directly related to metabolic acidosis.

69. D: Hyperventilation is associated with acidosis.

70. D: In respiratory acidosis the heart rate may be within normal limits or slow.

71. C: During respiratory alkalosis the patient most often hyperventilates and becomes flushed.

72. C: Pentoxifylline is used to treat peripheral vascular disease.

73. D: Bumex is a loop diuretic for long-term treatment of CHF.

74. C: Aldactone is a potassium-sparing diuretic.

75. C: Digoxin does not increase venous pressure.

76. C: Normal sinus rhythm is not usually noted when a client is digoxin toxic.

77. A: Muscle twitching is most often noted with hypernatremia.

78. A: Hypernatremia is associated with high blood pressure.

79. C: The digoxin level should be between 0.7 and 22 ng/mL. All other listed ranges are accurate.

80. C: Primidone should be 2 to 19 mcg/mL. All other listed ranges are accurate.

81. D: Carbamazepine levels should be 1.4 to 12 mcg/mL. All other listed ranges are accurate.

# How to Overcome Test Anxiety

Just the thought of taking a test is enough to make most people a little nervous. A test is an important event that can have a long-term impact on your future, so it's important to take it seriously and it's natural to feel anxious about performing well. But just because anxiety is normal, that doesn't mean that it's helpful in test taking, or that you should simply accept it as part of your life. Anxiety can have a variety of effects. These effects can be mild, like making you feel slightly nervous, or severe, like blocking your ability to focus or remember even a simple detail.

If you experience test anxiety—whether severe or mild—it's important to know how to beat it. To discover this, first you need to understand what causes test anxiety.

## Causes of Test Anxiety

While we often think of anxiety as an uncontrollable emotional state, it can actually be caused by simple, practical things. One of the most common causes of test anxiety is that a person does not feel adequately prepared for their test. This feeling can be the result of many different issues such as poor study habits or lack of organization, but the most common culprit is time management. Starting to study too late, failing to organize your study time to cover all of the material, or being distracted while you study will mean that you're not well prepared for the test. This may lead to cramming the night before, which will cause you to be physically and mentally exhausted for the test. Poor time management also contributes to feelings of stress, fear, and hopelessness as you realize you are not well prepared but don't know what to do about it.

Other times, test anxiety is not related to your preparation for the test but comes from unresolved fear. This may be a past failure on a test, or poor performance on tests in general. It may come from comparing yourself to others who seem to be performing better or from the stress of living up to expectations. Anxiety may be driven by fears of the future—how failure on this test would affect your educational and career goals. These fears are often completely irrational, but they can still negatively impact your test performance.

> **Review Video: 3 Reasons You Have Test Anxiety**
> Visit mometrix.com/academy and enter code: 428468

# Elements of Test Anxiety

As mentioned earlier, test anxiety is considered to be an emotional state, but it has physical and mental components as well. Sometimes you may not even realize that you are suffering from test anxiety until you notice the physical symptoms. These can include trembling hands, rapid heartbeat, sweating, nausea, and tense muscles. Extreme anxiety may lead to fainting or vomiting. Obviously, any of these symptoms can have a negative impact on testing. It is important to recognize them as soon as they begin to occur so that you can address the problem before it damages your performance.

> **Review Video: 3 Ways to Tell You Have Test Anxiety**
> Visit mometrix.com/academy and enter code: 927847

The mental components of test anxiety include trouble focusing and inability to remember learned information. During a test, your mind is on high alert, which can help you recall information and stay focused for an extended period of time. However, anxiety interferes with your mind's natural processes, causing you to blank out, even on the questions you know well. The strain of testing during anxiety makes it difficult to stay focused, especially on a test that may take several hours. Extreme anxiety can take a huge mental toll, making it difficult not only to recall test information but even to understand the test questions or pull your thoughts together.

> **Review Video: How Test Anxiety Affects Memory**
> Visit mometrix.com/academy and enter code: 609003

# Effects of Test Anxiety

Test anxiety is like a disease—if left untreated, it will get progressively worse. Anxiety leads to poor performance, and this reinforces the feelings of fear and failure, which in turn lead to poor performances on subsequent tests. It can grow from a mild nervousness to a crippling condition. If allowed to progress, test anxiety can have a big impact on your schooling, and consequently on your future.

Test anxiety can spread to other parts of your life. Anxiety on tests can become anxiety in any stressful situation, and blanking on a test can turn into panicking in a job situation. But fortunately, you don't have to let anxiety rule your testing and determine your grades. There are a number of relatively simple steps you can take to move past anxiety and function normally on a test and in the rest of life.

> **Review Video: How Test Anxiety Impacts Your Grades**
> Visit mometrix.com/academy and enter code: 939819

# Physical Steps for Beating Test Anxiety

While test anxiety is a serious problem, the good news is that it can be overcome. It doesn't have to control your ability to think and remember information. While it may take time, you can begin taking steps today to beat anxiety.

Just as your first hint that you may be struggling with anxiety comes from the physical symptoms, the first step to treating it is also physical. Rest is crucial for having a clear, strong mind. If you are tired, it is much easier to give in to anxiety. But if you establish good sleep habits, your body and mind will be ready to perform optimally, without the strain of exhaustion. Additionally, sleeping well helps you to retain information better, so you're more likely to recall the answers when you see the test questions.

Getting good sleep means more than going to bed on time. It's important to allow your brain time to relax. Take study breaks from time to time so it doesn't get overworked, and don't study right before bed. Take time to rest your mind before trying to rest your body, or you may find it difficult to fall asleep.

> **Review Video: The Importance of Sleep for Your Brain**
> Visit mometrix.com/academy and enter code: 319338

Along with sleep, other aspects of physical health are important in preparing for a test. Good nutrition is vital for good brain function. Sugary foods and drinks may give a burst of energy but this burst is followed by a crash, both physically and emotionally. Instead, fuel your body with protein and vitamin-rich foods.

Also, drink plenty of water. Dehydration can lead to headaches and exhaustion, especially if your brain is already under stress from the rigors of the test. Particularly if your test is a long one, drink water during the breaks. And if possible, take an energy-boosting snack to eat between sections.

> **Review Video: How Diet Can Affect your Mood**
> Visit mometrix.com/academy and enter code: 624317

Along with sleep and diet, a third important part of physical health is exercise. Maintaining a steady workout schedule is helpful, but even taking 5-minute study breaks to walk can help get your blood pumping faster and clear your head. Exercise also releases endorphins, which contribute to a positive feeling and can help combat test anxiety.

When you nurture your physical health, you are also contributing to your mental health. If your body is healthy, your mind is much more likely to be healthy as well. So take time to rest, nourish your body with healthy food and water, and get moving as much as possible. Taking these physical steps will make you stronger and more able to take the mental steps necessary to overcome test anxiety.

> **Review Video: How to Stay Healthy and Prevent Test Anxiety**
> Visit mometrix.com/academy and enter code: 877894

# Mental Steps for Beating Test Anxiety

Working on the mental side of test anxiety can be more challenging, but as with the physical side, there are clear steps you can take to overcome it. As mentioned earlier, test anxiety often stems from lack of preparation, so the obvious solution is to prepare for the test. Effective studying may be the most important weapon you have for beating test anxiety, but you can and should employ several other mental tools to combat fear.

First, boost your confidence by reminding yourself of past success—tests or projects that you aced. If you're putting as much effort into preparing for this test as you did for those, there's no reason you should expect to fail here. Work hard to prepare; then trust your preparation.

Second, surround yourself with encouraging people. It can be helpful to find a study group, but be sure that the people you're around will encourage a positive attitude. If you spend time with others who are anxious or cynical, this will only contribute to your own anxiety. Look for others who are motivated to study hard from a desire to succeed, not from a fear of failure.

Third, reward yourself. A test is physically and mentally tiring, even without anxiety, and it can be helpful to have something to look forward to. Plan an activity following the test, regardless of the outcome, such as going to a movie or getting ice cream.

When you are taking the test, if you find yourself beginning to feel anxious, remind yourself that you know the material. Visualize successfully completing the test. Then take a few deep, relaxing breaths and return to it. Work through the questions carefully but with confidence, knowing that you are capable of succeeding.

Developing a healthy mental approach to test taking will also aid in other areas of life. Test anxiety affects more than just the actual test—it can be damaging to your mental health and even contribute to depression. It's important to beat test anxiety before it becomes a problem for more than testing.

> **Review Video: Test Anxiety and Depression**
> Visit mometrix.com/academy and enter code: 904704

# Study Strategy

Being prepared for the test is necessary to combat anxiety, but what does being prepared look like? You may study for hours on end and still not feel prepared. What you need is a strategy for test prep. The next few pages outline our recommended steps to help you plan out and conquer the challenge of preparation.

## Step 1: Scope Out the Test

Learn everything you can about the format (multiple choice, essay, etc.) and what will be on the test. Gather any study materials, course outlines, or sample exams that may be available. Not only will this help you to prepare, but knowing what to expect can help to alleviate test anxiety.

## Step 2: Map Out the Material

Look through the textbook or study guide and make note of how many chapters or sections it has. Then divide these over the time you have. For example, if a book has 15 chapters and you have five days to study, you need to cover three chapters each day. Even better, if you have the time, leave an extra day at the end for overall review after you have gone through the material in depth.

If time is limited, you may need to prioritize the material. Look through it and make note of which sections you think you already have a good grasp on, and which need review. While you are studying, skim quickly through the familiar sections and take more time on the challenging parts. Write out your plan so you don't get lost as you go. Having a written plan also helps you feel more in control of the study, so anxiety is less likely to arise from feeling overwhelmed at the amount to cover. A sample plan may look like this:

- Day 1: Skim chapters 1–4, study chapter 5 (especially pages 31–33)
- Day 2: Study chapters 6–7, skim chapters 8–9
- Day 3: Skim chapter 10, study chapters 11–12 (especially pages 87–90)
- Day 4: Study chapters 13–15
- Day 5: Overall review (focus most on chapters 5, 6, and 12), take practice test

## Step 3: Gather Your Tools

Decide what study method works best for you. Do you prefer to highlight in the book as you study and then go back over the highlighted portions? Or do you type out notes of the important information? Or is it helpful to make flashcards that you can carry with you? Assemble the pens, index cards, highlighters, post-it notes, and any other materials you may need so you won't be distracted by getting up to find things while you study.

If you're having a hard time retaining the information or organizing your notes, experiment with different methods. For example, try color-coding by subject with colored pens, highlighters, or post-it notes. If you learn better by hearing, try recording yourself reading your notes so you can listen while in the car, working out, or simply sitting at your desk. Ask a friend to quiz you from your flashcards, or try teaching someone the material to solidify it in your mind.

## Step 4: Create Your Environment

It's important to avoid distractions while you study. This includes both the obvious distractions like visitors and the subtle distractions like an uncomfortable chair (or a too-comfortable couch that makes you want to fall asleep). Set up the best study environment possible: good lighting and a comfortable work area. If background music helps you focus, you may want to turn it on, but otherwise keep the room quiet. If you are using a computer to take notes, be sure you don't have any other windows open, especially applications like social media, games, or anything else that could distract you. Silence your phone and turn off notifications. Be sure to keep water close by so you stay hydrated while you study (but avoid unhealthy drinks and snacks).

Also, take into account the best time of day to study. Are you freshest first thing in the morning? Try to set aside some time then to work through the material. Is your mind clearer in the afternoon or evening? Schedule your study session then. Another method is to study at the same time of day that you will take the test, so that your brain gets used to working on the material at that time and will be ready to focus at test time.

## Step 5: Study!

Once you have done all the study preparation, it's time to settle into the actual studying. Sit down, take a few moments to settle your mind so you can focus, and begin to follow your study plan. Don't give in to distractions or let yourself procrastinate. This is your time to prepare so you'll be ready to fearlessly approach the test. Make the most of the time and stay focused.

Of course, you don't want to burn out. If you study too long you may find that you're not retaining the information very well. Take regular study breaks. For example, taking five minutes out of every hour to walk briskly, breathing deeply and swinging your arms, can help your mind stay fresh.

As you get to the end of each chapter or section, it's a good idea to do a quick review. Remind yourself of what you learned and work on any difficult parts. When you feel that you've mastered the material, move on to the next part. At the end of your study session, briefly skim through your notes again.

But while review is helpful, cramming last minute is NOT. If at all possible, work ahead so that you won't need to fit all your study into the last day. Cramming overloads your brain with more information than it can process and retain, and your tired mind may struggle to recall even previously learned information when it is overwhelmed with last-minute study. Also, the urgent nature of cramming and the stress placed on your brain contribute to anxiety. You'll be more likely to go to the test feeling unprepared and having trouble thinking clearly.

So don't cram, and don't stay up late before the test, even just to review your notes at a leisurely pace. Your brain needs rest more than it needs to go over the information again. In fact, plan to finish your studies by noon or early afternoon the day before the test. Give your brain the rest of the day to relax or focus on other things, and get a good night's sleep. Then you will be fresh for the test and better able to recall what you've studied.

## Step 6: Take a practice test

Many courses offer sample tests, either online or in the study materials. This is an excellent resource to check whether you have mastered the material, as well as to prepare for the test format and environment.

Check the test format ahead of time: the number of questions, the type (multiple choice, free response, etc.), and the time limit. Then create a plan for working through them. For example, if you have 30 minutes to take a 60-question test, your limit is 30 seconds per question. Spend less time on the questions you know well so that you can take more time on the difficult ones.

If you have time to take several practice tests, take the first one open book, with no time limit. Work through the questions at your own pace and make sure you fully understand them. Gradually work up to taking a test under test conditions: sit at a desk with all study materials put away and set a timer. Pace yourself to make sure you finish the test with time to spare and go back to check your answers if you have time.

After each test, check your answers. On the questions you missed, be sure you understand why you missed them. Did you misread the question (tests can use tricky wording)? Did you forget the information? Or was it something you hadn't learned? Go back and study any shaky areas that the practice tests reveal.

Taking these tests not only helps with your grade, but also aids in combating test anxiety. If you're already used to the test conditions, you're less likely to worry about it, and working through tests until you're scoring well gives you a confidence boost. Go through the practice tests until you feel comfortable, and then you can go into the test knowing that you're ready for it.

## Test Tips

On test day, you should be confident, knowing that you've prepared well and are ready to answer the questions. But aside from preparation, there are several test day strategies you can employ to maximize your performance.

First, as stated before, get a good night's sleep the night before the test (and for several nights before that, if possible). Go into the test with a fresh, alert mind rather than staying up late to study.

Try not to change too much about your normal routine on the day of the test. It's important to eat a nutritious breakfast, but if you normally don't eat breakfast at all, consider eating just a protein bar. If you're a coffee drinker, go ahead and have your normal coffee. Just make sure you time it so that the caffeine doesn't wear off right in the middle of your test. Avoid sugary beverages, and drink enough water to stay hydrated but not so much that you need a restroom break 10 minutes into the test. If your test isn't first thing in the morning, consider going for a walk or doing a light workout before the test to get your blood flowing.

Allow yourself enough time to get ready, and leave for the test with plenty of time to spare so you won't have the anxiety of scrambling to arrive in time. Another reason to be early is to select a good seat. It's helpful to sit away from doors and windows, which can be distracting. Find a good seat, get out your supplies, and settle your mind before the test begins.

When the test begins, start by going over the instructions carefully, even if you already know what to expect. Make sure you avoid any careless mistakes by following the directions.

Then begin working through the questions, pacing yourself as you've practiced. If you're not sure on an answer, don't spend too much time on it, and don't let it shake your confidence. Either skip it and come back later, or eliminate as many wrong answers as possible and guess among the remaining ones. Don't dwell on these questions as you continue—put them out of your mind and focus on what lies ahead.

Be sure to read all of the answer choices, even if you're sure the first one is the right answer. Sometimes you'll find a better one if you keep reading. But don't second-guess yourself if you do immediately know the answer. Your gut instinct is usually right. Don't let test anxiety rob you of the information you know.

If you have time at the end of the test (and if the test format allows), go back and review your answers. Be cautious about changing any, since your first instinct tends to be correct, but make sure you didn't misread any of the questions or accidentally mark the wrong answer choice. Look over any you skipped and make an educated guess.

At the end, leave the test feeling confident. You've done your best, so don't waste time worrying about your performance or wishing you could change anything. Instead, celebrate the successful completion of this test. And finally, use this test to learn how to deal with anxiety even better next time.

> **Review Video:** <u>5 Tips to Beat Test Anxiety</u>
> Visit mometrix.com/academy and enter code: 570656

## Important Qualification

Not all anxiety is created equal. If your test anxiety is causing major issues in your life beyond the classroom or testing center, or if you are experiencing troubling physical symptoms related to your anxiety, it may be a sign of a serious physiological or psychological condition. If this sounds like your situation, we strongly encourage you to seek professional help.

# Thank You

We at Mometrix would like to extend our heartfelt thanks to you, our friend and patron, for allowing us to play a part in your journey. It is a privilege to serve people from all walks of life who are unified in their commitment to building the best future they can for themselves.

The preparation you devote to these important testing milestones may be the most valuable educational opportunity you have for making a real difference in your life. We encourage you to put your heart into it—that feeling of succeeding, overcoming, and yes, conquering will be well worth the hours you've invested.

We want to hear your story, your struggles and your successes, and if you see any opportunities for us to improve our materials so we can help others even more effectively in the future, please share that with us as well. **The team at Mometrix would be absolutely thrilled to hear from you!** So please, send us an email (support@mometrix.com) and let's stay in touch.

If you'd like some additional help, check out these other resources we offer for your exam:

http://MometrixFlashcards.com/CRNA

# Additional Bonus Material

Due to our efforts to try to keep this book to a manageable length, we've created a link that will give you access to all of your additional bonus material.

Please visit **https://www.mometrix.com/bonus948/crna** to access the information.